VISUAL AIDS
FOR
PARAMEDICAL VOCABULARY

VISUAL AIDS
FOR
PARAMEDICAL VOCABULARY

By

J. E. SCHMIDT, M.D.

CHARLES C THOMAS • PUBLISHER

Springfield • Illinois • U.S.A.

Published and Distributed Throughout the World by
CHARLES C THOMAS • PUBLISHER
BANNERSTONE HOUSE
301-327 East Lawrence Avenue, Springfield, Illinois, U.S.A.

ISBN 0-398-02609-2
Library of Congress Catalog Card Number: 72-84149

Printed in the United States of America
W-2

INTRODUCTION

It is generally believed that the study of a technical vocabulary, such as the vocabulary of medicine, must of necessity be a dull and onerous task. The belief is well founded, for all books dealing with new terminologies, including foreign languages, basically do no more than offer lists of words that the student is expected to learn on the mere basis of a definition—without contextual aid—and then commit to memory by rote. The labor of such a method of learning is truly discouraging.

In this book the author departs from the old inquisitional format by presenting the words in a kind of "natural and painless wordbirth" that does away with the doldrums. The presentation is enlivened by visual aids in the form of 165 exceptionally vivid illustrations.

The format of this textbook is basically a simplified discussion of the medical subjects which by their nature involve the most useful medical terms, especially for the paramedical student and practitioner. Thus, the bulk of the book is devoted to a discussion of the following systems:

The Skeletal System
The Circulatory System
The Digestive System
The Urinary System
The Sensory System
The Muscular System
The Nervous System
The Respiratory System
The Reproductive System
The Endocrine System

Each chapter narrates the subject in an accurate but simplified manner, with the words to be learned appearing unobtrusively in the company of a pleasant context that obviates the need for a wearying effort at memorization. At the end of each chapter there is a list of words for review, as well as a commentary on derivation and allied matters. There are also exercises and stimulating questions.

There are also chapters on the sources of medical words and

on the "anatomy" of medical vocabulary. The latter gives considerable lexical detail about roots, stems, combining forms, prefixes, and suffixes, and explains how these elements are combined to form compound words. The book also contains a chapter discussing the human body as a whole and serving as a suitable introduction to the chapters on the various systems, which follow.

Finally, and perhaps above all, one should mention the *Visual Aids* feature consisting essentially of detailed line drawings. It may be a cliché, but it is certainly true that a medical illustration is worth a thousand words of definition and explanation. The visual aspect of a word not only helps in understanding the word but is also a great mnemonic aid. A word seen as a picture is a word remembered.

The illustrations in this book were originally published in the Attorneys' Dictionary of Medicine & Word Finder *(by this author) and in* Trauma, *and are reprinted through the permission of the copyright owner, Matthew Bender & Company, Inc.*

J.E.S.

OTHER BOOKS BY THE AUTHOR

English Speech for Foreign Physicians, Scientists, Students
English Idioms and Americanisms for Foreign Students, Professionals and Physicians
English Word Power for Physicians and Other Professionals
Medical Discoveries: Who and When
The Medical Lexicographer
Narcotics: Lingo and Lore
Paramedical Dictionary
Police Medical Dictionary
Practical Nurses' Medical Dictionary
Structural Units of Medical and Biological Terms

CONTENTS

Page

Introduction v

Acknowledgment vii

Chapter

I. The Sources of Medical Words 3

II. The Anatomy of Medical Vocabulary 5

III. Preliminary Considerations 10

IV. The Skeletal System 19

V. Body Directions or Positions 62

VI. The Muscular System 68

VII. The Circulatory System 77

VIII. The Nervous System 89

IX. The Digestive System 112

X. The Respiratory System 127

XI. The Urinary System 135

XII. The Reproductive System 141

XIII. The Auditory System 154

XIV. The Visual System 159

XV. The Endocrine System 167

XVI. Illustrations of Common Fractures 177

VISUAL AIDS
FOR
PARAMEDICAL VOCABULARY

Chapter I

THE SOURCES OF MEDICAL WORDS

MOST MEDICAL TERMS—more than 90 percent—are derived from Greek and Latin. A great number of these words have been in circulation for 2000 years or more, though not necessarily bearing the same definitions that they do now. Among the words that have been used for many centuries are the following: *alopecia* (baldness); *amblyopia* (dimness of vision); *anthrax; ascites* (accumulation of fluid in abdomen); *bronchus* (an air-conducting tube in the lung); *cholera; coccyx* (the lowest segment of the spine); *emphysema; hernia; meninges* (membranes covering brain); *mydriasis* (dilatation of the pupil); *nephritis* (inflammation of the kidney); *pus; skeleton; strabismus* (squint); *typhus.*

THE IMAGERY OF THE ANCIENT WORD MAKERS. In coining new words, the old neologists were greatly influenced by the names and forms of familiar objects, as fruits, vegetables, weapons, utensils, animals. Thus, they named the little tongue of flesh in the back of the mouth *uvula* because it reminded them of the grape, which is *uva* in Latin. The *streptococcus* suggested the berry, which is *kokkos* in Greek.

The *deltoid* muscle (a muscle of the shoulder) bears a resemblance to the Greek letter *delta,* hence the name. Another Greek letter, *sigma,* is responsible for the *sigmoid* portion of the colon (large intestine), because it has an S-like configuration.

A small bone of the wrist reminded the ancients of the *pea,* which is *pisum* in Latin; they named it *pisiform.* A *muscle* is from the Latin *musculus,* a little mouse. The snail-like structure of the inner ear is called *cochlea,* the word for *snail* in Greek.

Among the tools that influenced the word makers are the anvil (*incus* in Latin), which gave the name to one of the three bones of the middle ear, and the hammer (*malleus* in Latin), which suggested the name for another.

Then there are the weapons. *Xiphos,* the Greek for *sword,* is the name source of the *xiphoid process,* the lower part of the breastbone. The sheath of the sword, *vagina* in Latin, was an imaginative appellation for the female passage to the uterus. The shield, *thyreos* in Greek, is responsible for the *thyroid* gland.

WORDS BASED ON MEDICAL MISCONCEPTIONS. A small group of medical words bear the stigmas of medical misconceptions, although they are properly formed from classical structural units. Among these words are *melancholia, artery, pituitary, phlegmatic. Melancholia* is derived from the Greek *melas,* black, and *chole,* bile, and was so named because the physicians of the period believed that the unhappy emotional state was caused by the presence of black bile in the body. *Artery* is derived from the Greek *aer,* air, and *terein,* to keep or carry, because the ancient observers believed that the arteries carry air. The *pituitary* gland, derived from the Latin *pituitarius* (secreting phlegm), was so designated because it was believed to be responsible for the formation of mucus or phlegm in the nose.

SOURCES OTHER THAN LATIN AND GREEK. While the overwhelming majority of our medical terms are derived from Greek and Latin, the mainstream has a few minor tributaries. The Anglo-Saxons contributed the common terms used by both the medical practitioners and by the laity, such as *arm, bladder, finger, foot, hair, hand, head, heart, lung, neck, sick, swell.* The French language supplied *chancre, cretin, grippe, poison, tampon.* Arabic is the source of *alcohol, camphor, syrup, tartar,* and a few others.

A sprinkling of biological and scientific terms come from a variety of languages, as *borax* and *talc* (from Persian), *Fahrenheit* (German), *influenza* (Italian), *cough, litmus,* and *splint* (Dutch), *cascara* (Spanish).

Chapter II

THE ANATOMY OF MEDICAL VOCABULARY

ONLY A RELATIVELY small number of medical words are composed of single units; that is, of one word taken from Greek, Latin, French, or any other language. Most medical words are compound words, formed from two, three, or even more structural units, usually of Greek or Latin origin. For example, the word *cholecystitis* is a tripartite compound that can be dissected into the following three units: *chole* (bile), *cyst* (bladder), and *itis* (inflammation). *Cholecystitis,* therefore, means inflammation of the gall (or bile) bladder.

The units of which compound words are formed are known as *combining forms.* Each combining form is in turn derived from the base, the stem, or the root of a source language, usually Greek or Latin.

BASE, ROOT, STEM, AND OTHER STRUCTURAL UNITS. *Base* is a more general term, comprising *root* and *stem,* which may be defined as the residue of a compound word from which the inflectional appurtenances have been removed. In the word *biological, biolog* is the base. In *untapped, tap* is the base.

A *root* is the smallest linguistic particle common to a group of cognate words. It is the unreducible part of a *base.* In other functions, a root may be regarded as the linguistic unit to which prefixes, suffixes, or certain vowels are added to form an inflected or more complex word. Thus, *move* is the root of moved. *Possible* is the root of *impossible. Believe* is the root of *unbelievingly.*

A *stem* is a linguistic particle or unit usually consisting of a root and a vowel or consonant letter, and serving as the structure to which an inflectional form is added. In the Latin word *tendere* (to stretch), *tend* is the *stem, ten* is the *root, ere* is the *inflectional form,* and *d* is the *thematic letter* which converts the *root* into a *stem.*

A *prefix* is a simple linguistic structure, not used alone but having a definite meaning. It is attached to the beginning of a base, root, stem, or another prefix. In *untamed, un* is a prefix. In *unregenerate,* both *un* and *re* are prefixes, one attached to the other, and both attached to *generate*.

A *suffix* is linguistically similar to a prefix, but it is affixed to the end of a base, root, or stem. Many suffixes carry no specific ideas. In the word *applicable, able* is a suffix conveying the general concept of *capable of being* (in this case capable of being applied). The suffix *ary,* used to form nouns, designates a person employed as, or a thing used for, as in *apothecary, dictionary.*

HOW MEDICAL WORDS ARE FORMED

Simple words, i.e. words consisting of only one root or stem, are often taken *literatim* from Greek or Latin, as in the case of *abdomen* and *hernia.* Compound words, i.e. words consisting of two or more stems, are formed by the union of Greek or Latin words or their stems. Words consisting of one stem and a prefix or suffix may also be regarded as compound.

THE DERIVATION OF COMBINING FORMS. The classic words used to compound medical terms must first be modified in order to qualify them as suitable combining forms. The combining form, it will be remembered, is a base, root, or stem which may differ markedly from the more familiar lexical form of the word (the form that would be found in a Greek or Latin dictionary).

COMBINING FORMS FROM GREEK NOUNS. The combining form or stem of nouns ending in *a, e, as, es, os* or *on* is found by dropping these endings. In many other cases the combining form is derived not from the nominative case, as above, but from the genitive form, by dropping the terminal *os.* Still another group of combining forms are derived from both the nominative case and the genitive case (e.g. *hem*angioma, from the nominative case, and *hemato*cyst, from the genitive case).

COMBINING FORMS FROM LATIN NOUNS. The combining forms or stems of a large group of Latin nouns are found by dropping the terminal *us, um, a, u,* or *es* from the nominative singular.

The stems of another group of nouns are found by dropping the terminal *i* or *is* from the genitive case.

COMBINING FORMS FROM GREEK AND LATIN VERBS. A number of combining forms are derived from the past participle of Latin verbs and the future tense of Greek verbs. Most combining forms derived from Greek verbs are found by dropping the terminal *o, mai,* or *mi* from the present indicative, or the *ein, an, sthai,* or *nai* from the infinitive. Some combining forms derived from Latin verbs are found by dropping the terminal *eo, io, or,* or *o* of the present indicative, or the *are, ere,* or *ire* of the infinitive.

The past participles of Latin verbs yield the corresponding combining forms when the terminal *us* is deleted. The deleted *us* is often replaced by a silent *e,* as in *acute,* which is derived from *acutus.* The combining forms derived from present participles of Latin verbs end in *ant* or *ent.* They are found by dropping the terminal *is* of the genitive case. (The present participle is used as an adjective and is declined in the same way.)

HOW COMBINING FORMS ARE JOINED

Some compound words—words composed of two or more combining forms or stems—existed as such in ancient Greek or Latin and were admitted into the current medical vocabulary stream intact. Most compound words, however, were and are formed by joining two or more Greek or Latin stems in accordance with certain principles. When the stems are Greek, the first stem is joined with the following one by the interposition of a connecting vowel, usually an *o* or an *i.* In the case of Latin stems, the connecting vowel is most commonly an *o* or an *i,* but sometimes a *u.* These connecting vowels have no semantic significance. They are merely the mortar holding the structural units together. When the second stem begins with a vowel, the connecting vowel is dispensed with. If the second stem begins with a vowel while the first ends with one, the terminal vowel of the first stem is dropped, as in the case of *hemuresis,* derived from the Greek *haima* and *uresis.*

HOW PREFIXES ARE JOINED WITH STEMS

A Greek prefix ending in a vowel, and a stem beginning with a consonant may be joined simply, without additions, deletions, or alterations (example: *amphi*theater). When a Greek prefix ending in a vowel is joined to a stem beginning with a vowel, the final vowel of the prefix is dropped (example: *di*uretic—from *dia* and uretic). The prefix *peri* is an exception. It retains the terminal vowel, as in *peri*arterial (surrounding an artery). A Greek prefix ending in a consonant, and a stem beginning with a vowel may be joined by simple addition (example: *syn*arthrosis—a joint permitting no motion). When a Greek prefix ending in a consonant must be joined with a stem beginning with a consonant, the final consonant of the prefix undergoes a change. Thus, when the consonant of the prefix is an *n*, it becomes an *l* before an *l* (of the stem), as in *syllable* (*syn* plus *lambanein*); it becomes an *m* before an *m, p,* or *b,* as in *symmetry* (from *syn* plus *metron*); it is dropped before an *s,* as in *systole* (from *syn* and *stellein*).

Latin prefixes follow the same rules that govern Greek prefixes, explained above. When the prefix ends in a vowel, or the stem begins with a vowel, the prefix and stem are joined by simple addition. When the prefix ends with a consonant and the stem begins with a consonant, the terminal consonant of the prefix undergoes a change. As is the case with Greek prefixes, when the terminal consonant is an *n*, the *n* becomes an *l* before a following *l,* as in *illustrate* (from *in* and *lustrare*). It becomes an *m* before a following *m, p,* or *b,* as in *imbibe* (from *in* and *bibere*). It becomes an *r* before a following *r,* as in *ir*rational (*in* plus *rational*). In addition, Latin prefixes ending in *d, x,* and *b* permit the final consonant to be assimilated by and become the same as the following consonant (of the stem). Thus, *ad* before a *c* becomes *ac,* as in *ac*cede (from *ad* plus *cedere*); it becomes *af* before an *f,* as in *af*filiate (*ad* plus *filius*); and it becomes *at* before a *t,* as in *attune* (*ad* plus *tune*). Similarly, *ex* becomes *ef* before an *f,* as in *effect* (from *ex* plus *facere*), and *ob* becomes *oc* before a *c,* as in *oc*cur (*from ob* plus *currere*).

HOW SUFFIXES ARE JOINED WITH STEMS

A suffix is usually attached directly to the stem or combining form which it follows, without the insertion of a connecting vowel. When the simple union of stem and suffix would result in a combination of sounds that is difficult to pronounce, certain changes are made in the ending of the stem. Many suffixes are used to convert one part of speech into another, as a verb into a noun. Thus, the Greek verb *charattein* (to ingrave) is changed into a noun by the addition of the suffix *ter* to the stem, producing the familiar word *character*. In a similar manner, the verb *crystallize* is derived from the Greek noun *krystallos* (crystal) by the addition of the suffix *ize*. Similar techniques are used in Latin.

Chapter III

PRELIMINARY CONSIDERATIONS

THE STUDY OF THE vocabulary of medicine would be extremely dull and laborious without at least a modicum of understanding of the human body and its functions. To provide the student with the necessary background in the anatomy, physiology, and pathology, of the human body, this book is divided into several sections, each dealing with a group of organs or a system of the body and with the vocabulary related to the structures, functions, and disorders of the particular system.

Even before this—before taking up the various subdivisions of the body, it will be profitable to discuss the body as a whole and to draw attention to the similarities between the human or animal body and a modern architectural structure, especially a modern home.

THE HUMAN BODY AS A WHOLE

Because the basic structural units of the body are microscopic in size, it is not obvious to the naked eye that the body is composed of tiny building blocks known as *cells*. A cell may be visualized as a brick of a brick building, or any other structural unit, such as a cinder block. The number of cells is almost inestimable—there are billions of them.

KINDS OF CELL. Cells are not all of the same kind, shape, or nature. They vary enormously, depending on the structure or tissue of which they are a part. In several ways they are indeed similar. A typical cell of a soft tissue may be envisioned as a tiny globule of living fluid contained within a very delicate *membrane*, somewhat resembling a small grape (the skin of which is roughly comparable to the membrane). The living fluid contained within the membrane is called *cytoplasm* (the plasm or *protoplasm* of the cell). The cytoplasm may be envisioned as the soft, semifluid contents of a grape.

STRUCTURE OF A CELL. The unit structure of the body, the cell, is thus composed of a tiny, literally microscopic sac containing the living fluid known as *cytoplasm*. In or near the center of the sac of cytoplasm is a structure called the *nucleus*. It, too, is surrounded by a delicate membrane. The nucleus is a very important part of the cell; the cell cannot live without it. Just as the cell contains a nucleus, the nucleus contains a tiny structure known as the *nucleolus,* which is particularly important in the reproduction of the cell. Another important constituent of the nucleus is the *chromatin,* a material which stains deeply with basic dyes. During the reproduction process of a cell, the chromatin gives rise to the *chromosomes,* rod-shaped bodies which carry the *genes.* The genes are concerned with the transmission of hereditary characteristics. The fluid and the formed substances within the nucleus are known as the *nucleoplasm.* Both nucleoplasm and cytoplasm are also known by the more general term *protoplasm.*

THE REPRODUCTION OF CELLS. The complex process by which a cell divides to form two new cells is called *mitosis.* The process is divided into four stages: *prophase, metaphase, anaphase,* and

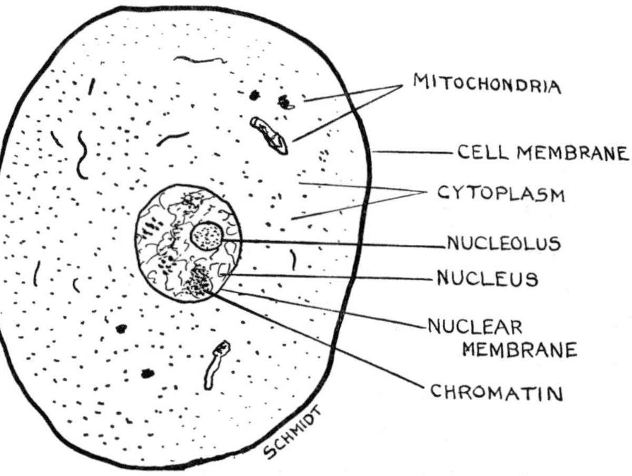

Figure 1. Diagram of a typical cell.

telophase. During the *prophase,* the chromatin of the nucleus becomes concentrated in the form of a tangled thread, the *spireme,* while the nuclear membrane disappears. A little later the thread or spireme breaks up into short segments, the *chromosomes.* At the same time two star-like structures appear in the cytoplasm of the cell outside the nucleus, one opposite the other, as are the poles of the earth. The "poles" seem to produce lines of force or attraction which may be visualized as the meridian lines of the earth.

During the second stage, the *metaphase,* the chromosomes formed during the prophase arrange themselves along what may be regarded as the equator of the cell (similar to the equator of the earth). Each chromosome then splits lengthwise into two halves. This ends the second stage.

During the third stage, the *anaphase,* the split chromosomes separate into two groups, each daughter chromosome facing one of the poles mentioned above. Then each daughter chromosome begins to move along a meridian line toward the pole nearest to it. Finally, all daughter chromosomes traveling toward one of the poles form a compact group at the pole or star-like structure. The other group of daughter chromosomes form a similar compact mass at the opposite pole. In this way, half of each original chromosome (i.e. daughter chromosome) is now located at one pole of the cell while the other half is situated at the opposite pole. Each pole has the same number of daughter chromosomes, the number being equal to the original number of chromosomes in the cell. This ends the third stage.

In the fourth stage, the *telophase,* a membrane (a nuclear membrane) forms around each group of daughter chromosomes at the two poles. The young chromosomes then lose their individuality and fuse into one mass of chromatin, one at each pole. The original cell now seems to have two nuclei, one at each pole. Soon the cytoplasm at the equator or "waist" of the cell begins to constrict, forming a structure similar to an hourglass. Finally the separation becomes complete, and we now have two cells, complete with nuclei, in place of the one.

THE CHARACTERISTICS OF PROTOPLASM. Protoplasm is the basic

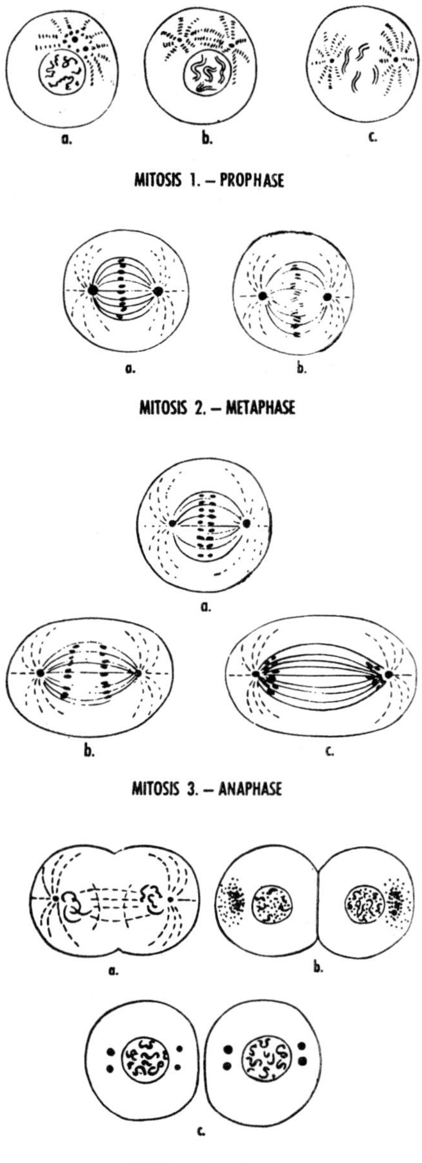

Figure 2. The four stages or phases in the process of division of a cell.

living substance of cells, tissues, organs, and the body as a whole. From a chemical point of view, it is not a remarkable substance. It is composed of ordinary materials that are part of the things we see around us every day. What is extraordinary about protoplasm is not its composition (water, mineral elements, sugars, fats) but its characteristics of *irritability, motility, metabolism, growth,* and *reproduction*—all of which add up to life. We can produce a substance chemically and physically similar to or identical with protoplasm, but we cannot endow it with life.

Irritability: The property of protoplasm that we call irritability is manifested by the ability of living matter to react in some manner to a stimulus or irritation. The most reactive or irritable cells of the body are the nerve cells, although muscles or muscle cells and protoplasm in general are also irritable to a smaller extent.

Motility: Protoplasm as such and certain cells have the power of movement. The protoplasm within cells exhibits motion. The best example of such movement is found in the *ameba,* a microscropic single-cell animal which consists of a tiny sac of protoplasm. The ameba causes its protoplasm to bulge out in fingerlike extensions from the main body (as fingers from the hand), and then pours all of the protoplasm of the cell into one of these extensions or "fingers," thus achieving a change in position. Certain white blood cells move in the same manner.

Metabolism: By "metabolism" is meant the chemical and physical processes taking place in the protoplasm of cells for the purpose of releasing energy needed for the vital functions of the organism and the cell itself. The processes comprise those by which digested food is assimilated and built up into protoplasm, and those by which protoplasm is used and broken down into simpler substances or waste matter. The process of building up is known more specifically as *anabolism;* the process of breaking down, as *catabolism.*

Growth: The fourth characteristic of living matter is growth, the process by which a cell or an organism attains full size and maturity. Growth is also involved in the repair of damaged tissue or protoplasm.

Reproduction: None of the characteristics of living matter is more important than reproduction, the process by which cells or organisms give rise to other cells or organisms of the same kind. Individual cells and simple organisms reproduce by the process of mitosis described above. Human beings and other complex animals reproduce by the union of specialized reproductive cells, the female *ovum* or egg cell and the male *spermatozoon* or sperm cell.

TISSUES

THE NATURE OF A TISSUE. It was stated above that the cell is the basic unit of structure of the body, comparable to the brick of a brick building. The next larger structure of the body is a *tissue*. A tissue is a large group of cells joined or bound together for the purpose of performing a particular function. Muscle is a tissue; fat is also a tissue; so is bone, cartilage, and nerve.

CONNECTIVE TISSUE. The several types of tissue will be discussed later, in dealing with the various systems of the body. *Connective tissue* is a tissue which binds and holds other tissues together. It may be regarded as a kind of "mortar." For example, the skin is attached to the underlying structures by connective tissue. Every organ of the body is held in place by connective tissue. There are several kinds of connective tissue, each kind suited for a particular function and each kind composed of cells that make it fit for its specialized function. When a tissue must be tough and unyielding, it is composed mainly of fibers and is called *fibrous tissue*. When its function is best served by resilience, it is made of elastic matter and is called *elastic tissue*.

EPITHELIAL TISSUE. Another tissue which has a more or less subservient role is *epithelium* or epithelial tissue. Epithelium is a sheet-like tissue which covers the outer surfaces of the body and lines the inner surfaces. It forms the outer layer or covering of the skin as well as the most superficial layer of the membranes lining the inner surfaces of the body, such as the bladder. Epithelium may be compared to a layer of wallpaper or a coat of paint.

ORGANS AND SYSTEMS

STRUCTURE AND FUNCTION OF AN ORGAN. An *organ* is generally a complex structure, more complex than a tissue, performing a special function. A typical organ, like the liver, is composed of many types of cell and several kinds of tissue. A simple organ may be composed of only one kind of tissue, such as a small gland. All structures of the body are intended to perform some sort of function, but structures that support or bring about motion are not regarded as organs. Thus, a muscle is not an organ. The function of an organ is more subtle or specialized, such as secretion, digestion, or conversion of one substance into another. One may compare a tissue to the floor of a dwelling or to the plaster on a wall, but an organ is more like an air conditioner or a furnace, which performs a complex function.

What is a *system?* With regard to the body, a *system* is composed of an organ or organs and certain supporting structures of lesser complexity, all of which work together to perform one of the more important bodily functions, such as digestion or excretion. Thus, the kidneys, the ureters, the bladder, and the urethra form the urinary system. The chief systems of the body are as follows:

1. The skeletal system.
2. The muscular system.
3. The circulatory system.
4. The nervous system.
5. The digestive system.
6. The respiratory system.
7. The urinary system.
8. The reproductive system.
9. The endocrine system.

THE BODY CAVITIES

THE MAJOR AND MINOR CAVITIES. The spaces within the body are known as *cavities*. The minor or smaller cavities are the spaces within certain bones, especially the bones of the face. These are known as *sinuses*. The interior of the nose is called the nasal cavity; the mouth is the oral cavity. The major cavities are divided into two groups: the dorsal or back cavities, and the ventral or front cavities.

The Dorsal Cavities: The dorsal cavities (which may be regarded as one continuous cavity) are composed of the *cranial cavity* and the *vertebral cavity*. The cranial cavity is the space within the skull which contains the brain. The vertebral cavity is situated within the spinal column. It contains the spinal cord.

The Ventral Cavities: The ventral cavities comprise the *thoracic cavity*, the *abdominal cavity*, and the *pelvic cavity*. The abdominal cavity is situated within the abdomen and contains the various abdominal organs—the liver, stomach, intestine. It is continuous with (i.e. not separated from) the pelvic cavity or pelvis, which contains the bladder, the rectum, etc. The thoracic or chest cavity contains the lungs and the heart. It is separated from the abdominal cavity by a dome-shaped sheet of muscular tissue known as the *diaphragm*. The movement of the diaphragm, up and down, aids in respiration or breathing. The thoracic cavity may be regarded as consisting of the central *pericardial* cavity—containing the heart, and the two lateral or side cavities, the *pleural* cavities—containing the lungs.

ABDOMINAL REGIONS

In order to facilitate the descriptive location of the abdominal organs, the anterior surface of the abdomen is divided into nine regions by four intersecting lines, two vertical and two horizontal. The three upper regions, from left to right, are the *left hypochondriac, epigastric,* and *right hypochrondriac*. The three middle regions, from left to right, are the *left lumbar, umbilical,* and *right lumbar*. The three lower regions are the *left iliac, hypogastric,* and *right iliac*. The iliac regions are also known as *inguinal* regions.

VOCABULARY REVIEW

Define the following terms on the basis of the preceding discussion. Determine the pronunciation with the aid of a medical dictionary.

ameba
anabolism
anaphase
catabolism
cavity
cell
chromatin
chromosome
cytoplasm
gene
irritability
membrane
metabolism
metaphase
mitosis
motility
nucleolus
nucleoplasm
nucleus
organ
ovum
prophase
protoplasm
reproduction
spireme
system
telophase
tissue

VOCABULARY EXERCISE

Using a standard medical dictionary, find the combining forms entering into the formation of the following words:

anabolism
anaphase
catabolism
chromosome
cytoplasm
metabolism
metaphase
nucleoplasm
prophase
protoplasm
reproduction
telophase

Indicate the meaning of the following prefixes:

ana-
cata-
ir-
meta-
proto-
telo-

List the plural form of each of the following words:

ameba
nucleolus
nucelus
ovum

Chapter IV

THE SKELETAL SYSTEM

THE FUNCTION OF BONES. The main function of the bones, collectively known as the *skeleton,* is to provide a framework for the soft tissues of the body. In other words, the skeleton provides support and gives shape to the body. In this respect it is similar to the steel framework of a large building or the wooden framework of an ordinary house. The skeleton also provides points of attachment for muscles, and thereby affords the mechanism for motion. In addition to these, the bones in certain parts of the body form a protective housing for such delicate structures as the brain and the eyeball, and those bones which contain marrow produce red blood cells, some white blood cells, and blood platelets.

STRUCTURE OF BONES. Although bones are hardened by deposits of calcium, they are living tissues or organs. Every bone is covered by a membrane known as *periosteum.* The periosteum is composed of two layers. The outer layer carries blood vessels and nerves; the inner layer is concerned with the formation of new bone. A more delicate membrane, the *endosteum,* lines the interior surface of the bones which have a central marrow cavity.

Bones may be classified as long bones, short bones, and flat bones. The bone of the thigh is a typical long bone. One of the bones of a finger or toe is an example of a short bone. The bones of the skull are more or less flat bones, containing numerous cavities known as *sinuses.* An opening into a bone for the passage of blood vessels and nerves is called a *foramen.*

Each end of a long bone, as that of the thigh or arm, is called *epiphysis.* The shaft between the ends is known as *diaphysis.* In early life, the shaft or diaphysis is not firmly united with the epiphyses (plural of epiphysis) but is attached to the ends by a layer of cartilage. This cartilage or gristle is the place where growth in length takes place. When full growth is completed, the cartilage is converted into bone, and the line of union between diaphysis and epiphysis is known as *epiphyseal line.* Completion of growth usually occurs between the ages of 18 and 21.

With regard to density of structure, there are two kinds of bone: *compact* and *cancellous* or spongy. The exterior of all bones is composed of compact bone. The epiphyses of long bones are composed of spongy bone covered by a thin layer of compact bone. The shaft or diaphysis is composed almost entirely of compact bone. The bones of the skull, i.e. the flat bones, have two layers of compact bone (an external and an internal layer) and, sandwiched between the two, a layer of spongy or cancellous bone.

BONE MARROW. There are two kinds of marrow, red and yellow. Red marrow is found in the spongy bone of the epiphyses of long bones, in the *sternum* or breastbone, in the ribs, in the vertebrae, and in the flat bones of the skull. Yellow marrow is found in the spaces or medullary cavities of long bones. Red blood cells and some white blood cells are formed in red bone marrow.

PROJECTIONS AND DEPRESSIONS OF BONES. A *condyle* is a smooth, rounded eminence on the end of a bone which enters into the formation of a joint with another bone. The bone of the thigh has prominent condyles. A *crest* is an elevation in the form of a ridge. A *foramen* is an opening into, or a passage through, a bone—also, occasionally, an opening in a soft tissue. A *fossa* is a depression, hollow, or pit. A *head,* with reference to a bone, is the enlarged end. A *meatus* is the opening to a passage or canal. A *process* is an extension or projection from a bone (or from the cell of a nerve). A *sinus* is a cavity within a bone, especially a bone of the face, but the term is also applied to certain channels conveying blood. A *spine* (or spinous process) is a sharp bony projection, as of a vertebra. The term is also applied to the backbone or vertebral column. A *sulcus* is a groove or furrow in a bone or a soft tissue such as the brain. A *trochanter* is a bony projection, especially the *greater trochanter* or the *lesser trochanter* on the upper end of the bone of the thigh. A *tubercle* is a rough, rounded outgrowth on a bone, of normal origin. It is also a small mass of soft tissue, as in tuberculosis. A *tuberosity* is a large rounded projection on a bone.

JOINTS OR ARTICULATIONS

The region at which bones are attached to each other is known as a *joint* or *articulation.*

Types of Joint. Classified on the basis of movement, there are three kinds of joint. The first is that kind in which there is no motion at all, as in the bones of the skull. The second kind of joint allows a slight degree of motion, as is the case between the vertebrae of the spine. The third type of joint allows free motion, as in the case of the hip joint.

The freely movable joints are of several different kinds. The ball-and-socket kind of joint, as in the hip and shoulder, allows the maximum amount of motion. A pivot joint, as in the case of the elbow, permits a rotary movement. The hinge joint permits movement in one plane, an example of which is the knee joint.

Ligaments and Bursae. The ends of bones entering into the formation of a joint are usually held in place by strong bands of fibrous tissue known as *ligaments.* In the structure of some joints, the ends of the bones are covered by plates of cartilage. These are called *articular cartilages.* Some joints have spaces or potential spaces which are surrounded by a *synovial membrane* and filled by *synovial fluid.* A *bursa* is a small sac filled with fluid which acts as a cushion in places where motion is likely to cause friction. Bursae are found between ligaments or tendons and bones, between muscles and bones, etc.

BONES OF THE SKULL

The skull is divided into two parts, the *cranium* and the *face.* The cranium is the part of the skull containing the brain. The remaining part of the skull comprises the facial bones.

THE CRANIAL BONES. The cranium is composed of two paired bones (i.e. left and right bones bearing the same name) and four single bones. The single bones are the *frontal* bone, the *occipital* bone, the *sphenoid* bone, and the *ethmoid* bone. The frontal bone forms the forehead and the greater part of the roof of the orbits or eye sockets. The occipital bone forms the back part of the cranium. It contains a large opening, the *foramen magnum,* for the passage of the spinal cord. The sphenoid bone forms the central part of the base or floor of the cranium. In front of it are the frontal and ethmoid bones; in back, the occipital bone. The ethmoid bone is located in the front part of the base or floor of the cranium, between the two eye sockets.

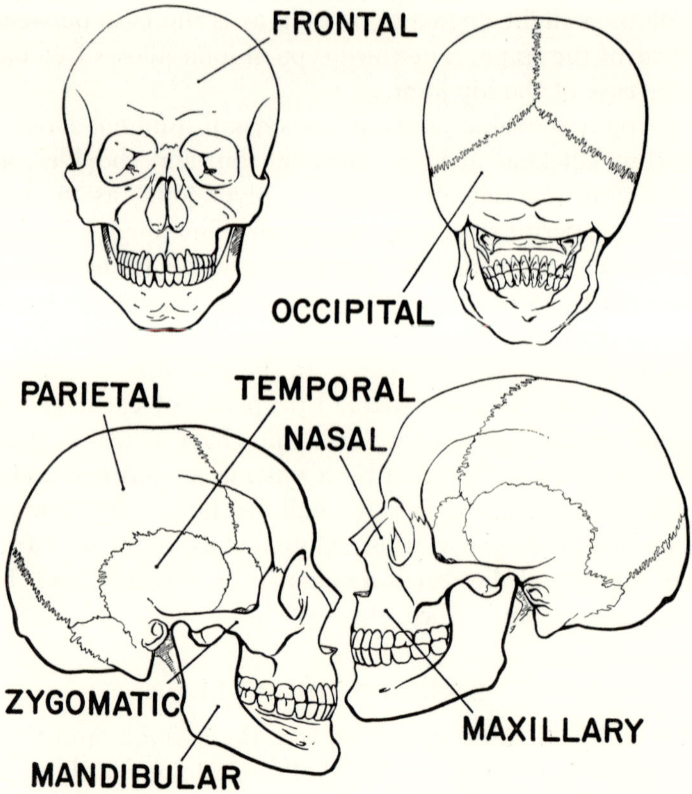

Figure 3. The front, back, and side views of the skull, showing the principal bones of the cranium and face.

The paired bones of the cranium are the right and left *parietal* bones and the right and left *temporal* bones. The two parietal bones are situated at the top of the cranium between the frontal bone and the occipital bone. The two bones meet in the midline (at the top of the head) and form the *sagittal suture.* Each of the two temporal bones is situated at the side of the cranium—one on the right side, the other on the left. The upper border of each bone forms a suture with the lower border of the corresponding parietal bone. The external surface of each temporal bone is marked by the *external acoustic meatus,* a canal which extends from the external ear to the *tympanic membrane* or eardrum.

THE BONES OF THE FACE. The facial bones are composed of six paired bones and two single bones. The paired bones are the *maxilla,* the *palatine* bones, the *zygomatic* bones, the *lacrimal* bones, the inferior *turbinates* or *conchae,* and the *nasal* bones. The single bones are the *vomer* and the *mandible* (lower jawbone). The maxilla is composed of two halves, a right and a left, fused in the midline of the face. Each half shares in the formation of the floor of the orbit, the walls of the nasal cavities, and the roof of the mouth. The palatine bones, a right and a left, are united in the midline of the mouth and form the back part of the roof of the mouth. The zygomatic bones form the prominences of the cheeks. The lacrimal bones contribute to the formation of the walls of the orbits or eye sockets. The inferior turbinates, one in each nostril, form horizontal projections upon the wall of the nose. The nasal bones form the upper part of the bridge of the nose. The vomer forms the lower back part of the *septum* of the nose (the "partition" which divides the interior of the nose into two chambers). The mandible or bone of the lower jaw consists of a horizontal portion, known as the *body,* and a perpendicular portion, known as the *rami* (singular *ramus*), extending from the back of the *body* to the side of the skull. The body of the mandible forms the chin and provides support for the teeth. The upper border or ridge of the body of the mandible, which contains the *alveoli* (singular *alveolus*) or openings for the teeth, is the *alveolar process.*

The *hyoid* bone is a small horseshoe-shaped bone situated

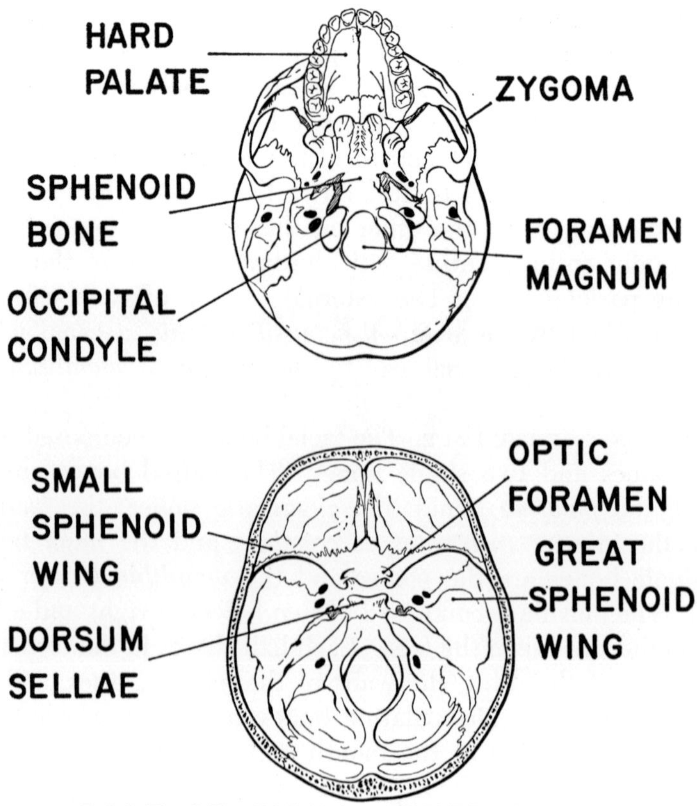

BASE OF SKULL, INNER SURFACE

Figure 4. Upper diagram shows the underside or base of the skull as seen from below. Hard palate is the roof of the mouth. Foramen magnum transmits the spinal cord. The occipital condyles form joints with the atlas, the first vertebra. The lower diagram shows the base of the skull as seen from the inside and from above.

below and behind the mandible. The muscles of the tongue are attached to it.

Four bones of the skull contain cavities known as *sinuses* or *antra* (singular *antrum*). These are the maxillary, frontal, ethmoid, and sphenoid sinuses, named after the bones in which they are found. The sinuses are lined by mucous membrane and drain into the nose.

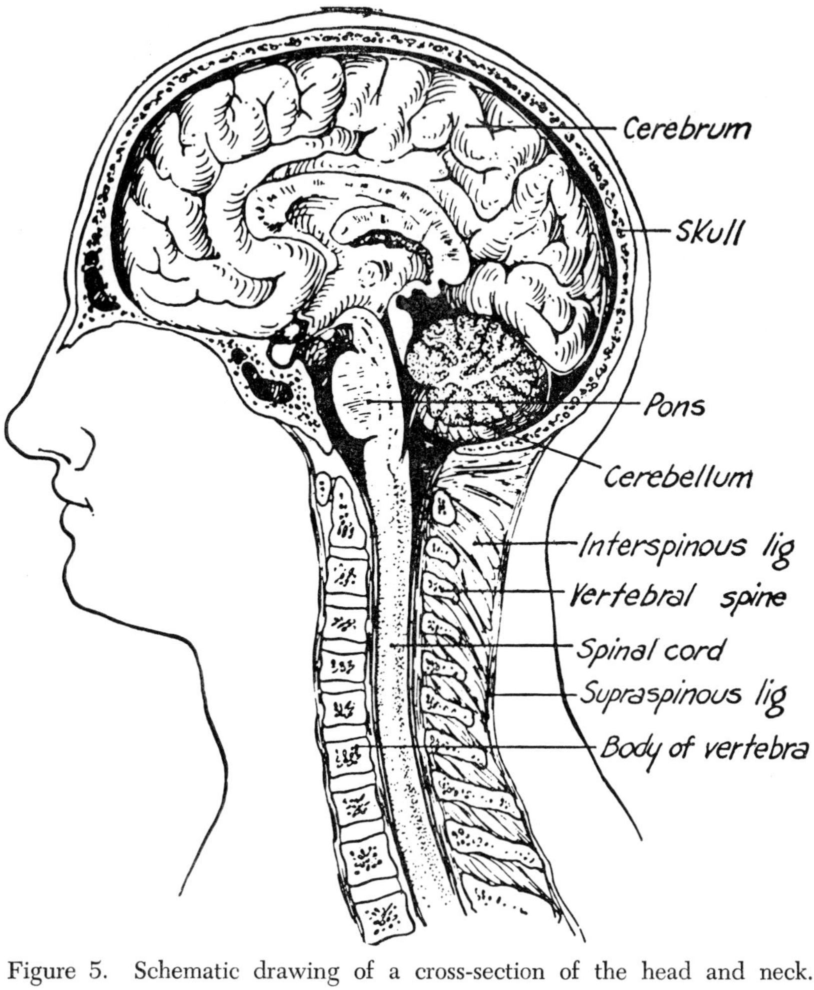

Figure 5. Schematic drawing of a cross-section of the head and neck.

VOCABULARY LESSON

On the basis of the preceding discussion, define the following terms. Determine the pronunciation of each word with the aid of a medical dictionary.

acoustic meatus	alveolus	cancellous
alveolar process	antra	concha
alveoli	antrum	condyle

cranium
crest
diaphysis
endosteum
epiphyseal line
epiphysis
ethmoid bone
foramen
foramen magnum
fossa
frontal bone
head
hyoid
lacrimal bones
ligament
mandible
maxilla
meatus
nasal bones
occipital bone
palatine bones
parietal bones
periosteum
process
rami
ramus
sagittal suture
septum
sinus
skeleton
sphenoid bone
spine
sternum
sulcus
synovial fluid
synovial membrane
temporal bones
trochanter
tubercle
tuberosity
turbinate
vomer
zygomatic bones

VOCABULARY EXERCISE

Using a standard medical dictionary, find the component parts, i.e. the combining forms, of the following words:

diaphysis
endosteum
epiphyseal
periosteum

What is the singular of the following words?

alveoli
antra
rami

Give the plural form of the following words:

concha
cranium
diaphysis
epiphysis
foramen
fossa
maxilla
septum
sternum
sulcus

BONES OF THE TRUNK

THE VERTEBRAL COLUMN. The *spine, spinal column,* or *vertebral column* is a hollow and flexible bony structure extending from the underside of the skull above to the lower border of the hip bones in the back. Its hollow contains the *spinal cord,* a cable-like structure of nerves making contact between the brain and the various parts of the body. The spine is not a single structure but a composite of 33 smaller bones called *vertebrae* (singular *vertebra*).

THE VERTEBRAE. Although the vertebrae are constructed on a common plan, they differ somewhat in size and detail, depending on their location within the spine. On the basis of their location, the vertebrae are divided into several groups. The seven vertebrae immediately below the skull are the *cervical* or neck vertebrae. The first vertebra, which supports the skull, is called the *atlas.* The vertebra below the atlas is the *axis.* The vertebrae *8* through *12* are the *thoracic* or chest vertebrae. They give support to the

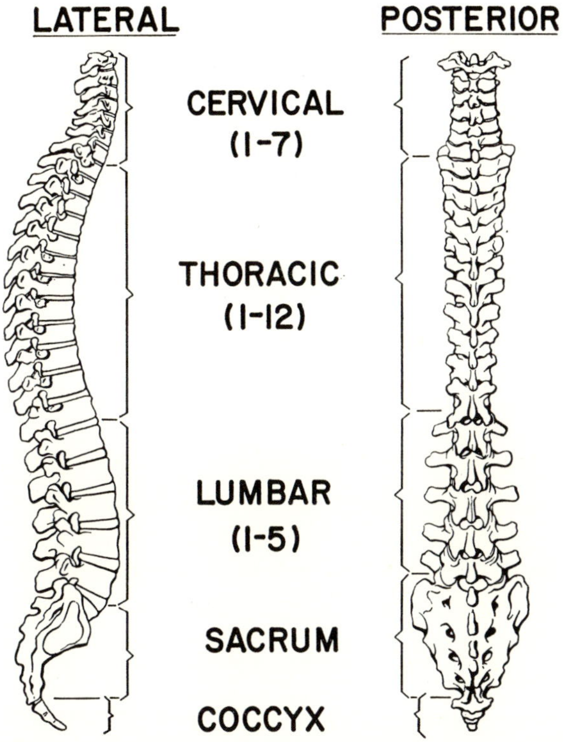

Figure 6. Lateral and posterior views of the spine or vertebral column, showing the several segments into which it is divided.

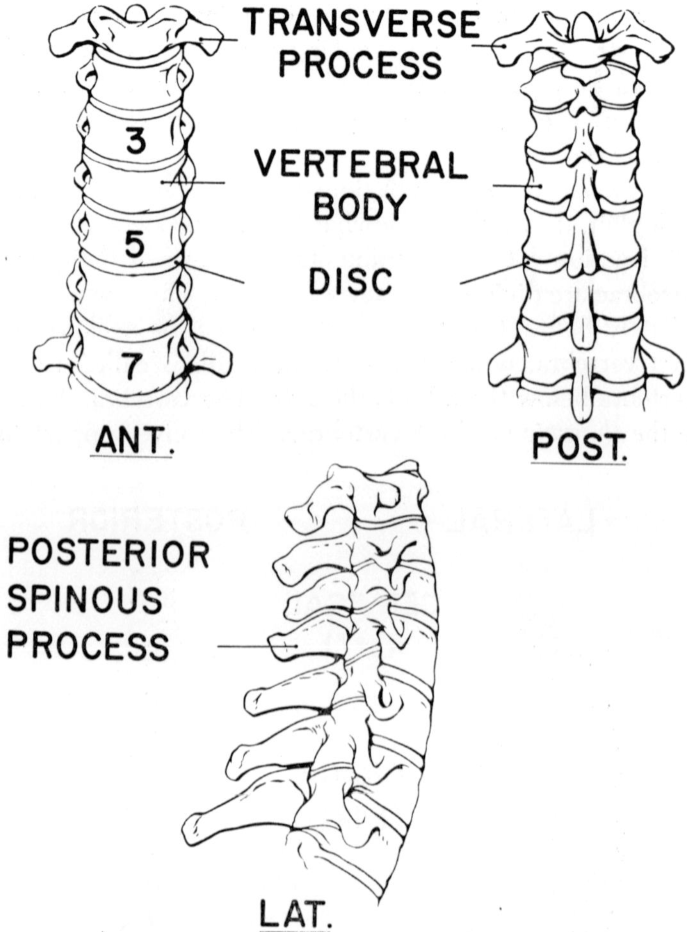

Figure 7. Anterior, posterior, and lateral views of the cervical or neck vertebrae.

ribs. The next five vertebrae are the *lumbar* or loin vertebrae. The cervical, thoracic, and lumbar vertebrae are distinct structures separated from each other by plates of cartilage called *intervertebral disks.* However, the next five vertebrae, the *sacral* vertebrae, are fused and form a solid bone, the *sacrum.* The last four vertebrae are not fully developed and are fused to form a single small bone, the *coccyx.* While the vertebrae have a similar structure varying somewhat in detail, a thoracic vertebra is regarded as a typical vertebra best exhibiting its various features.

A TYPICAL VERTEBRA. The front part of a vertebra is composed of a solid block of bone, *the body.* Extending backward from the body are two plates of bone, the *pedicles,* one on each side of the central opening of the vertebra, the *vertebral foramen* (which contributes to the formation of the canal housing the spinal cord). Extending backward from the pedicles and completing the bony wall around the vertebral foramen are the two (right and left) bony plates known as the *laminae* (singular *lamina*). The two laminae are fused in the back and from the region of junction extends a sturdy bony projection, the *spinous process* of the vertebra. From the region approximately midway between the spinous process and the body extends another bony projection, one on each side, the *transverse process.* There are, in addition, four smaller bony projections, two on each side, the *superior*

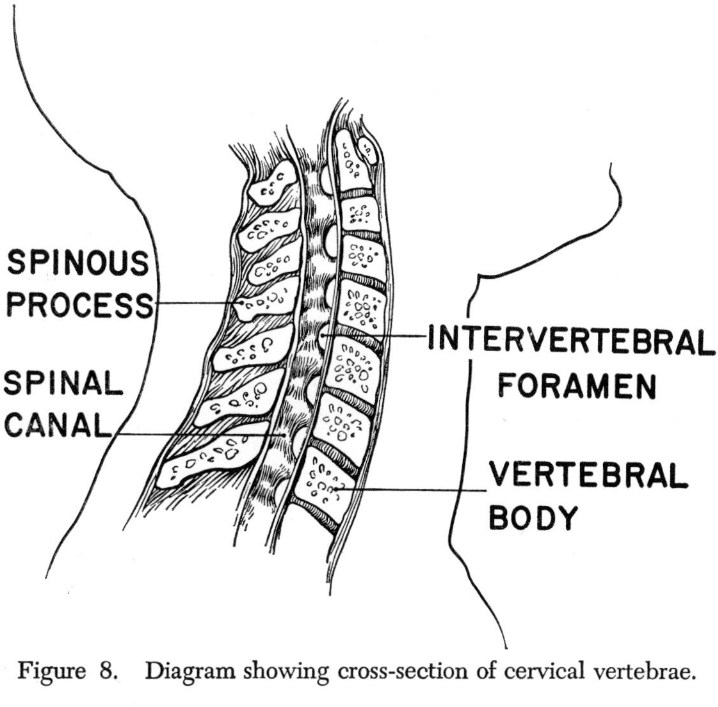

Figure 8. Diagram showing cross-section of cervical vertebrae.

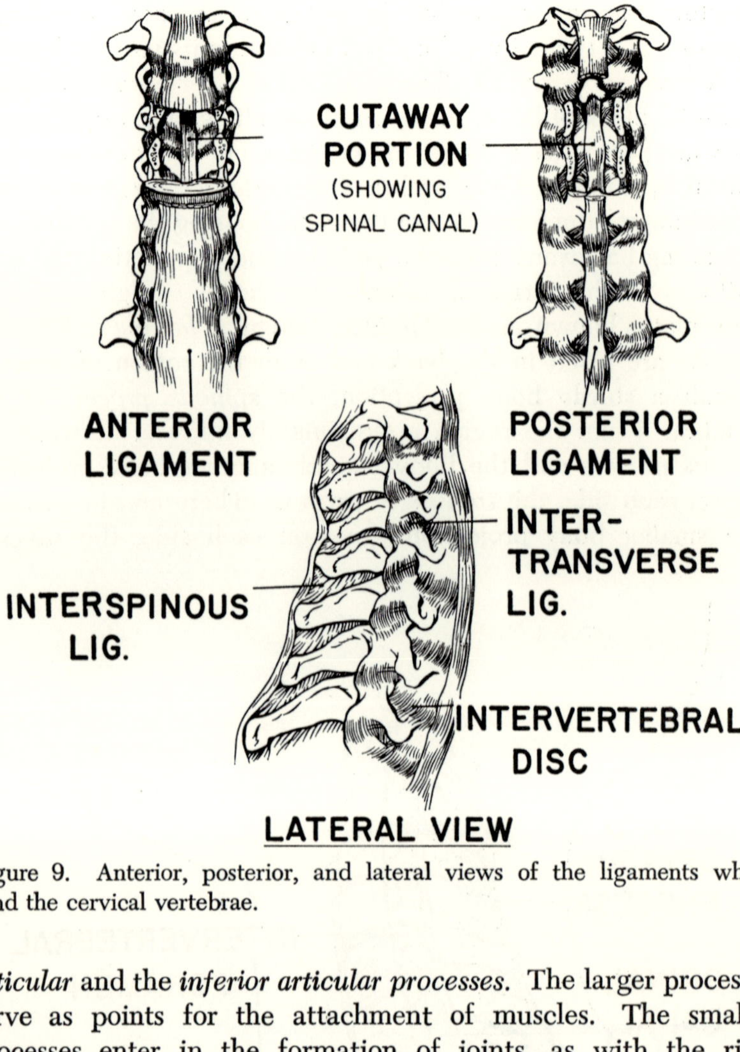

Figure 9. Anterior, posterior, and lateral views of the ligaments which bind the cervical vertebrae.

articular and the *inferior articular processes.* The larger processes serve as points for the attachment of muscles. The smaller processes enter in the formation of joints, as with the ribs.

BONES OF THE THORAX. The *thorax* or chest is a bony cage filled in and covered by muscles and other soft tissues. The bones which enter into the formation of the cage are the *thoracic vertebrae,* the *ribs,* and the *sternum.* The thorax is more or less cone-shaped, with the broad base below.

There are 24 ribs, 12 on each side of the chest. They may be visualized as the hoops of a barrel. Each rib is connected in the

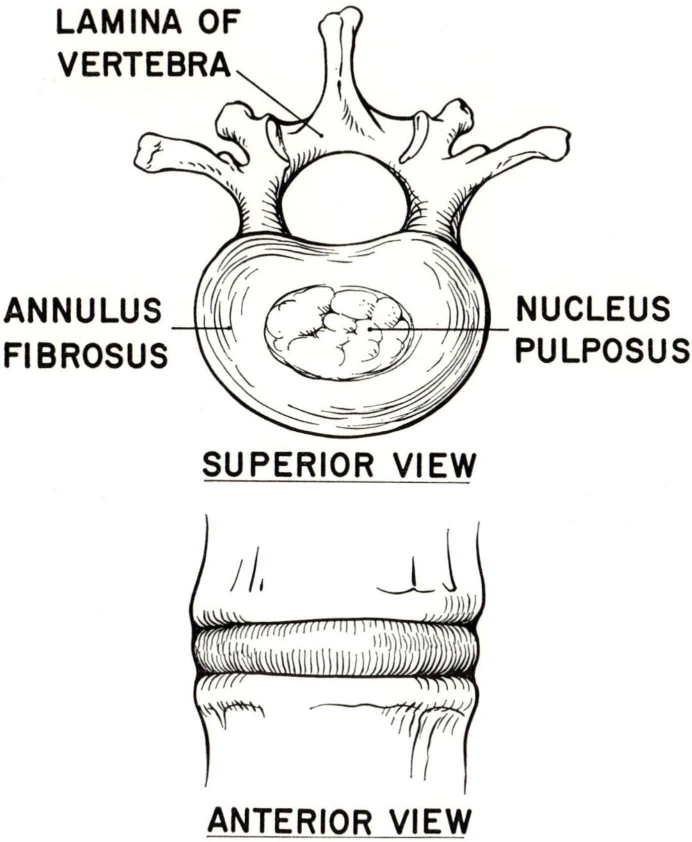

Figure 10. Anterior and superior views of an intervertebral disk, a structure frequently subject to trauma.

back to the vertebral column. The first seven pairs of ribs are attached in front to the sternum through the medium of a piece of cartilage, the *costal cartilage,* which is interposed between the front end of the rib and the sternum. These ribs are known as the "true" ribs. The next three pairs of ribs are attached to one another in front through their costal cartilages and then join the costal cartilage of the seventh rib. The last two pairs of ribs are free in front and are termed "floating" ribs.

The sternum or breastbone is composed of three parts. The upper segment is called the *manubrium* (because of its fancied

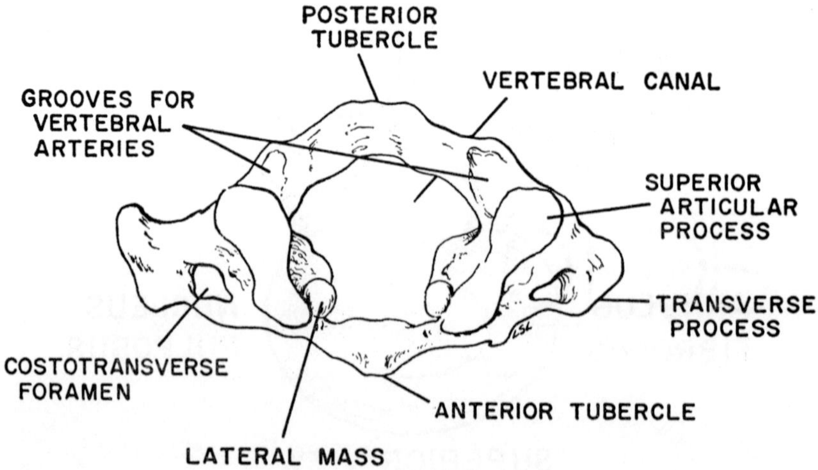

Figure 11. An anterior view of the atlas or first cervical vertebra, which supports the skull.

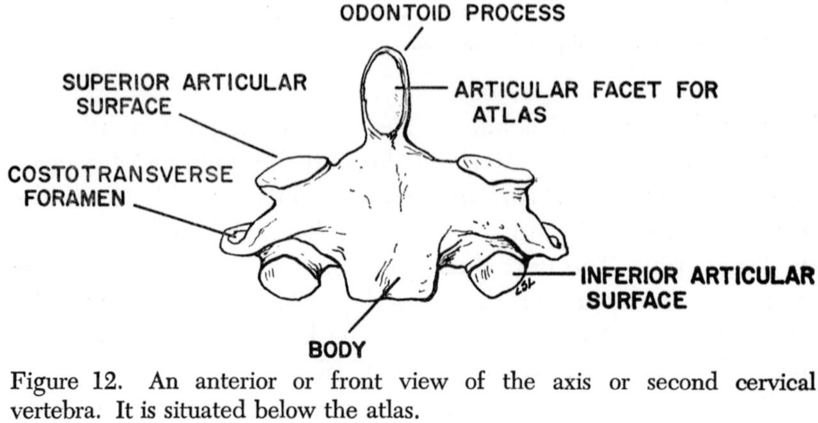

Figure 12. An anterior or front view of the axis or second cervical vertebra. It is situated below the atlas.

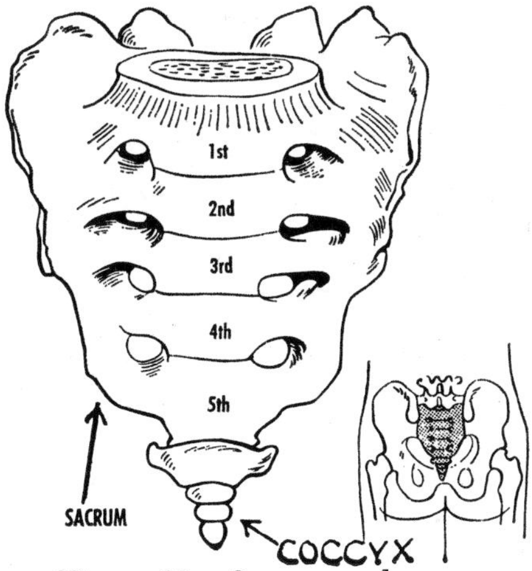

Figure 13. Sacrum and coccyx, the fused segments of the lower portion of the vertebral column.

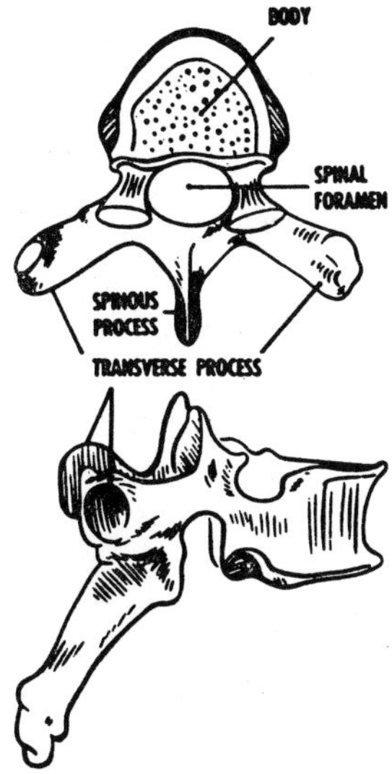

Figure 14. Superior and lateral views of a thoracic or chest vertebra showing the processes and the spinal or vertebral foramen which contains the spinal cord.

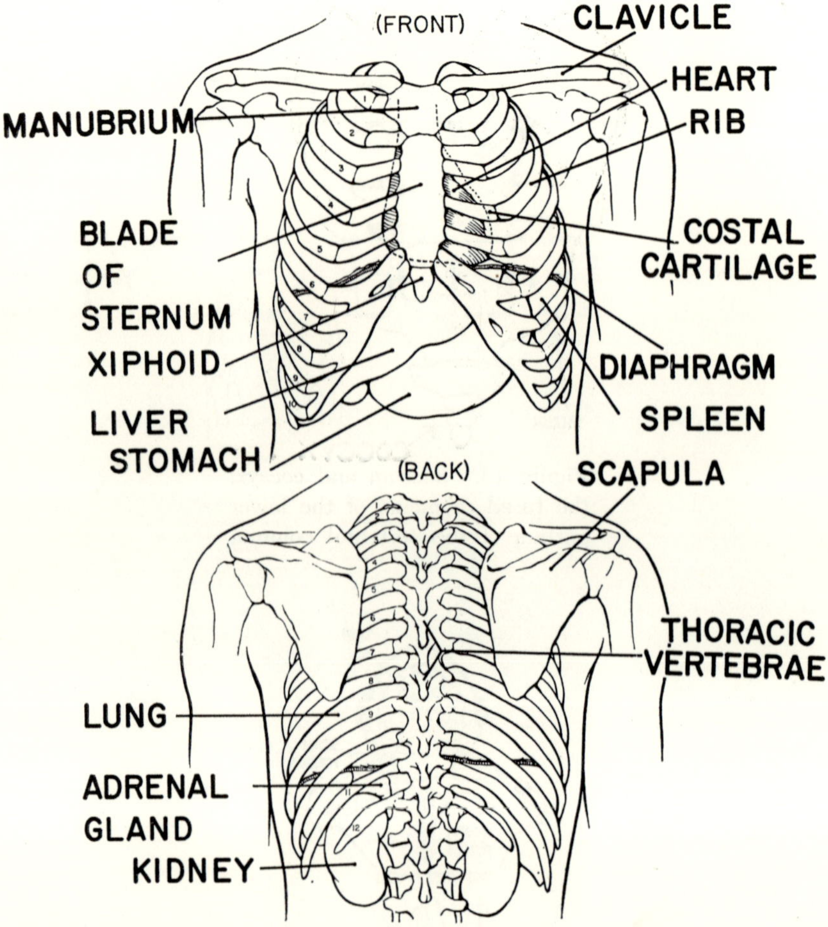

Figure 15. Front and back views of the rib cage or chest bones. Note position of organs with relation to the ribs.

resemblance to the handle of a sword). The middle segment is the *gladiolus*. The lower segment is the *xiphoid* (or *ensiform*) process.

The thorax contains and protects the heart, the lungs, the esophagus, the great blood vessels, and other structures.

Bones of the Pelvis. The pelvis, situated at the lower end of the trunk, is composed of two *innominate bones*, a right and a left, and the *sacrum*. It is a circular structure resembling a basin

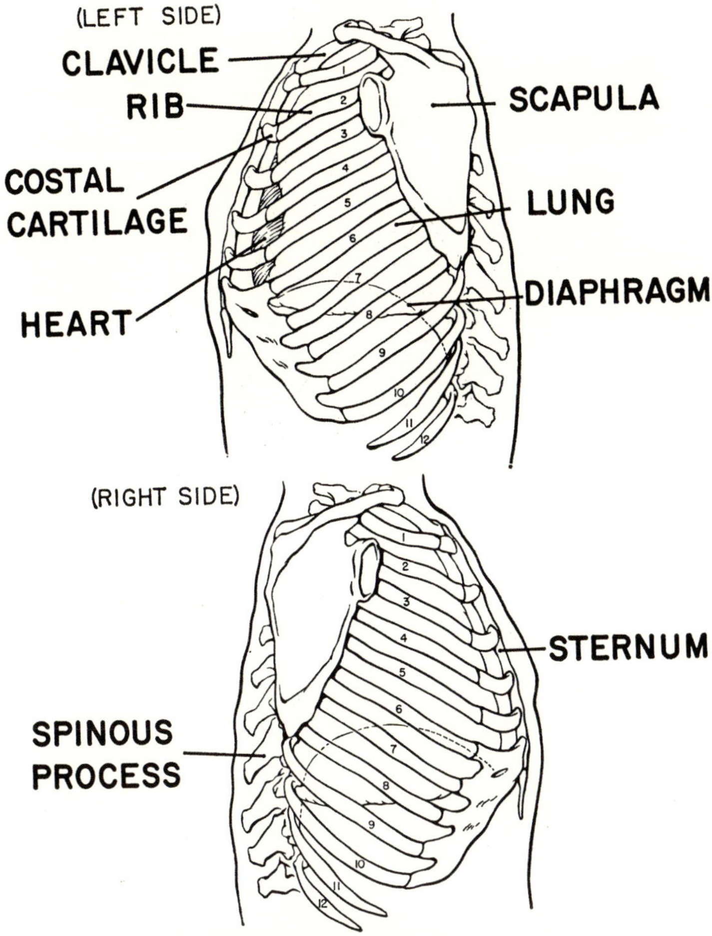

Figure 16. Left and right side views of the rib cage. Note position of heart and diaphragm.

or the upper part of a funnel. The junction of the innominate bones in front is known as the *symphysis pubis.* The two bones do not meet in the back, but are joined by the sacrum. Each innominate bone is composed of three smaller bones, the *ilium* (which is the largest and is regarded as the hip), the *ischium,* and the *pubis.* A rounded depression on the outer surface of each innominate bone, the *acetabulum,* acts as a socket for the upper end of the thigh bone. Through the medium of the sacrum

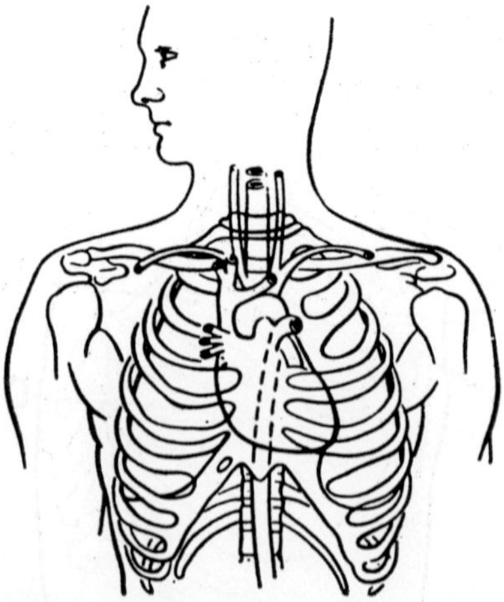

Figure 17. Diagram of rib cage showing position of heart in relation to sternum and ribs.

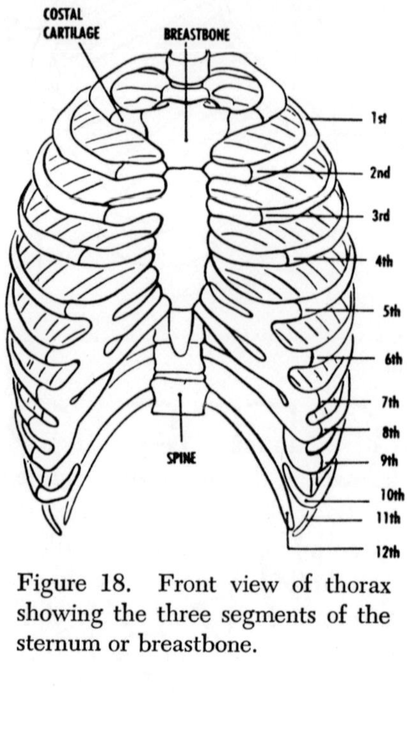

Figure 18. Front view of thorax showing the three segments of the sternum or breastbone.

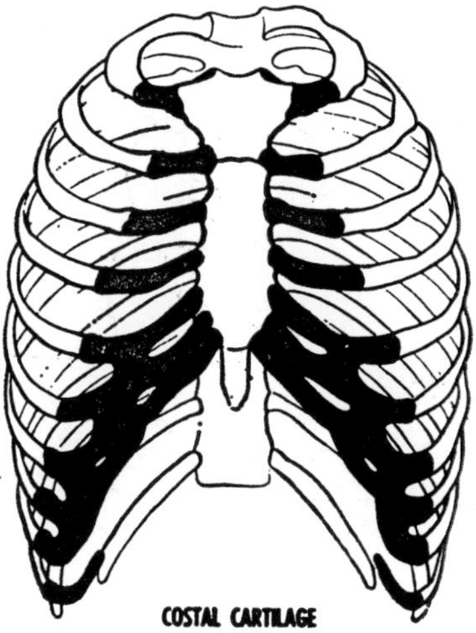

Figure 19. Front view of thorax or rib cage showing the costal cartilages (in black) by which the ribs are attached.

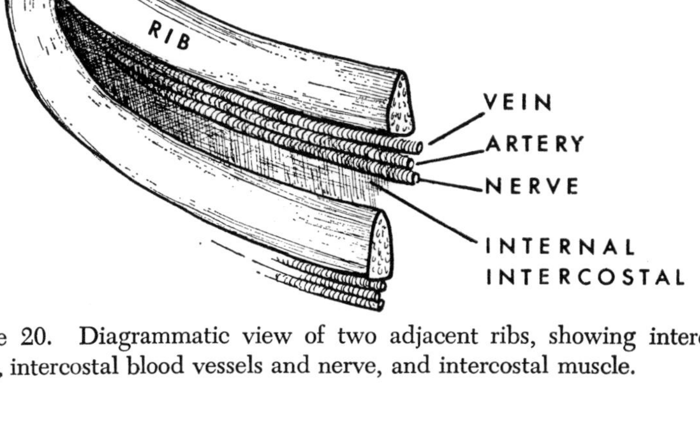

Figure 20. Diagrammatic view of two adjacent ribs, showing intercostal space, intercostal blood vessels and nerve, and intercostal muscle.

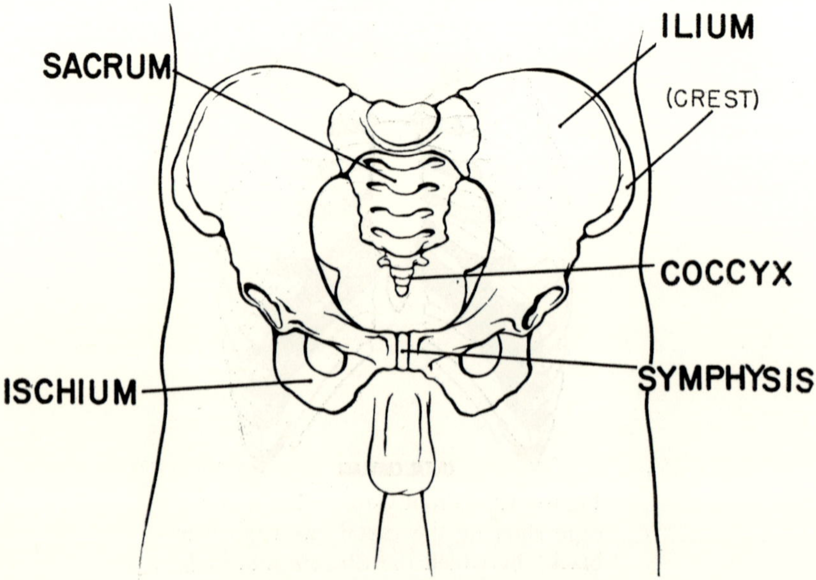

Figure 21. Front view of male pelvis.

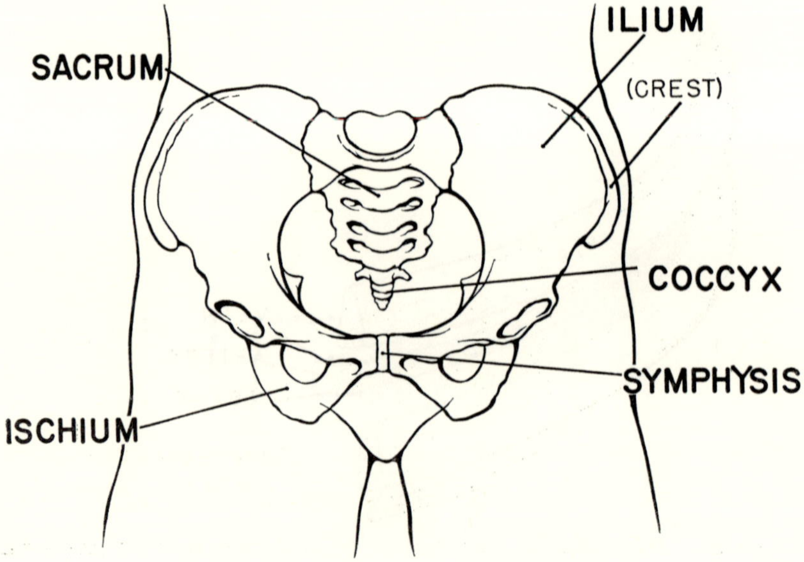

Figure 22. Front view of female pelvis.

the pelvis provides support for the spine while it is itself supported by the lower extremities. The interior of the pelvis is the *pelvic cavity,* which contains the bladder, the rectum, and the uterus. A woman's pelvis is relatively larger and wider than a man's.

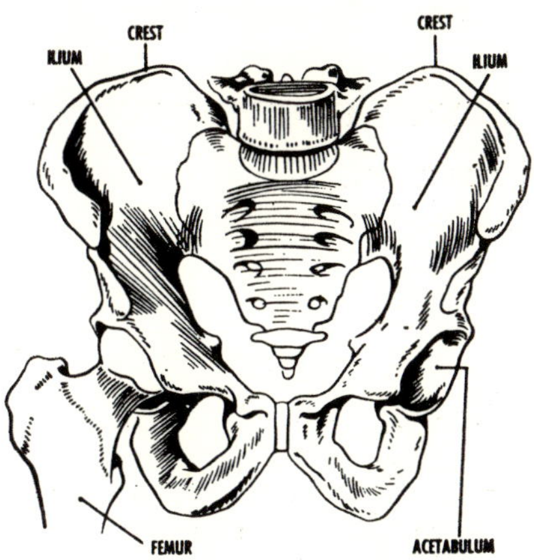

Figure 23. Bones of hip joint: the femur and innominate bone.

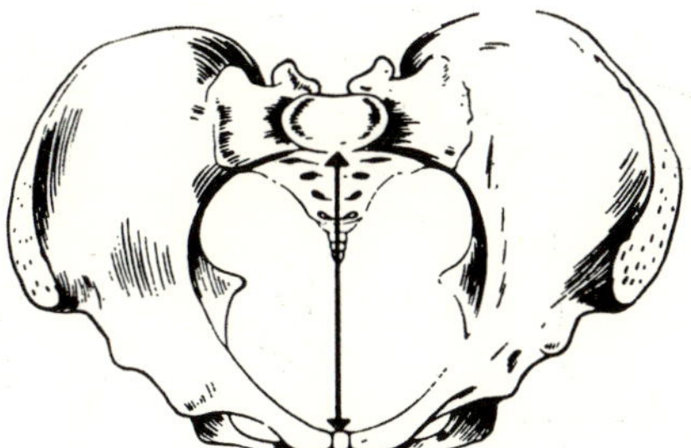

Figure 24. The anteroposterior diameter of the female pelvis.

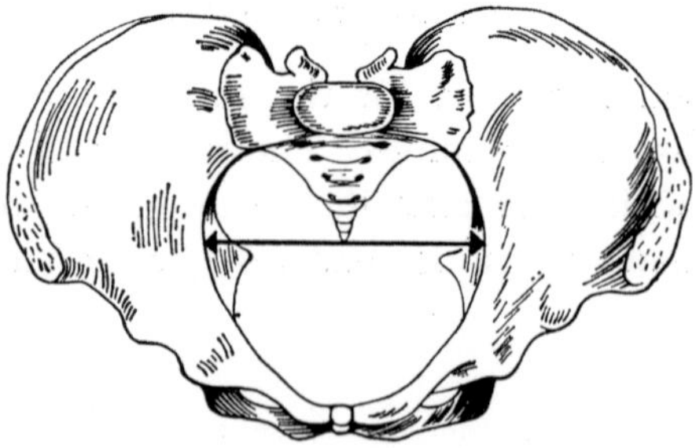

Figure 25. Transverse diameter of the female pelvis.

BONES OF THE EXTREMITIES

THE UPPER EXTREMITY. The upper extremity comprises the shoulder, the arm, the forearm, and the hand.

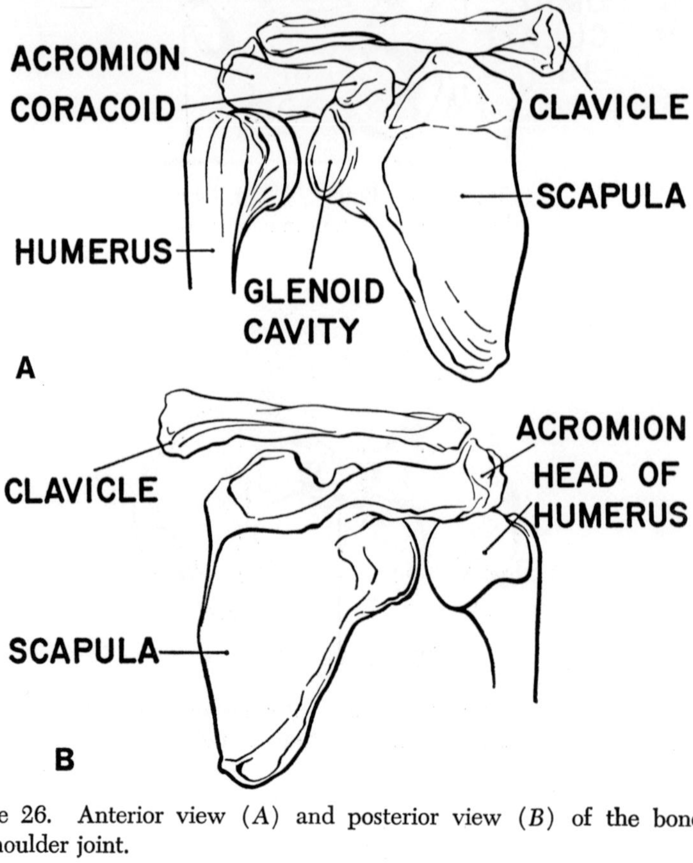

Figure 26. Anterior view (*A*) and posterior view (*B*) of the bones of the shoulder joint.

The Shoulder: The shoulder is composed of the *shoulder girdle* and the upper end of the bone of the upper arm (i.e. the humerus). The shoulder girdle is formed by the *clavicles* (collarbones) and the *scapulas* (shoulder blades). The clavicle is a slender bone extending horizontally from the tip of the shoulder to the manubrium of the sternum, to which it is attached. The scapula is a flat triangular bone situated with the base upward opposite the clavicle, i.e. in the back of the thorax. It is attached to the outer end of the clavicle at the *acromion process*, a bony outgrowth. Another bony outgrowth of the scapula is the *coracoid process*, situated in front of the acromion. Somewhat below and between these processes is a shallow depression, the *glenoid cavity*, which receives the rounded upper end of the bone of the arm to form the shoulder joint.

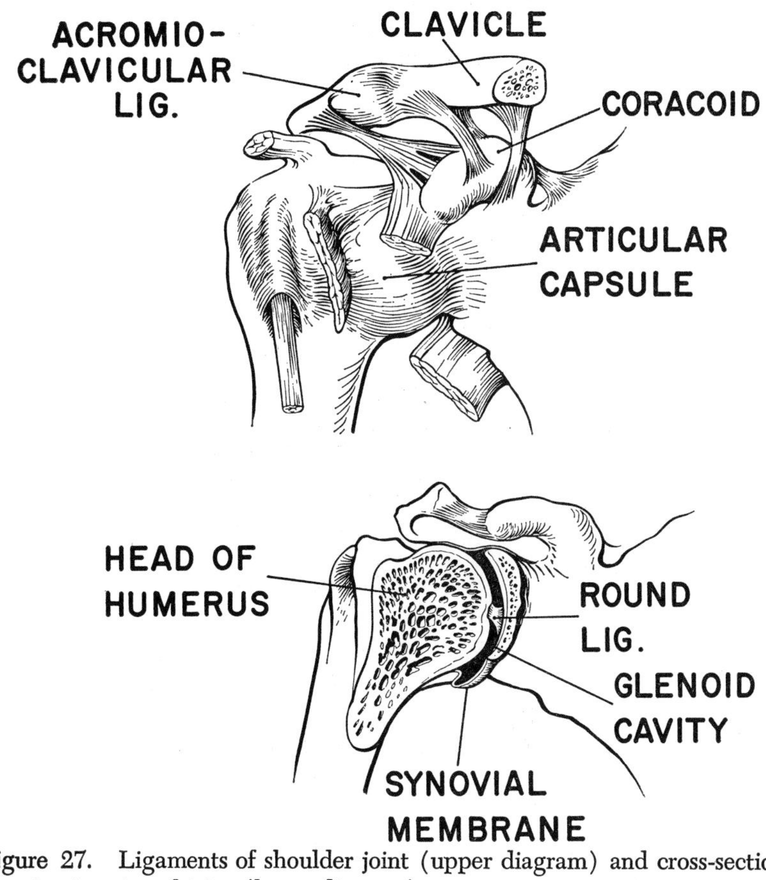

Figure 27. Ligaments of shoulder joint (upper diagram) and cross-section showing interior of joint (lower diagram).

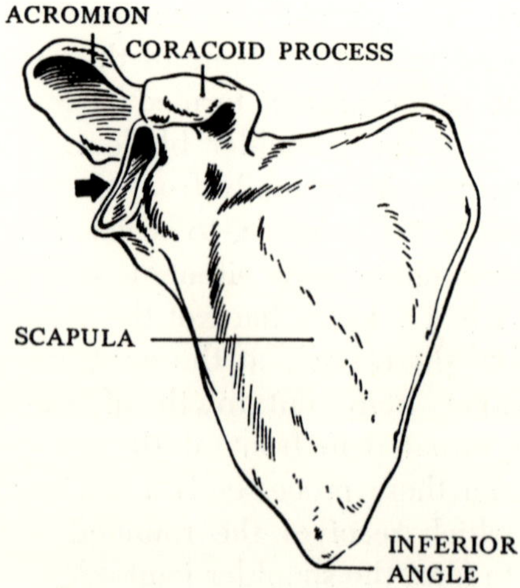

Figure 28. The scapula or shoulder blade showing acromion and coracoid process.

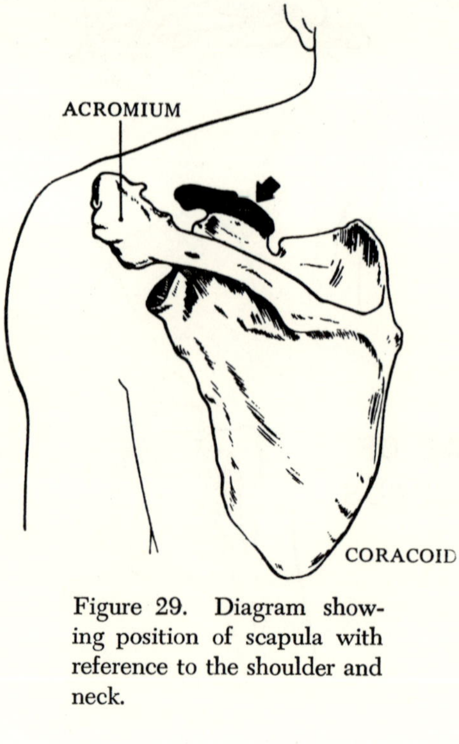

Figure 29. Diagram showing position of scapula with reference to the shoulder and neck.

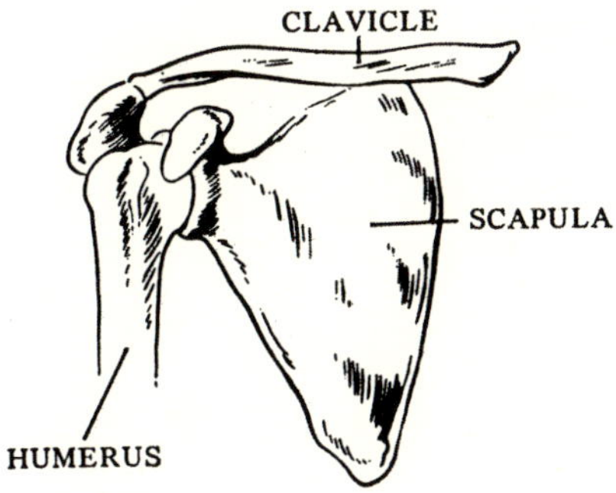

Figure 30. The bones of the shoulder girdle.

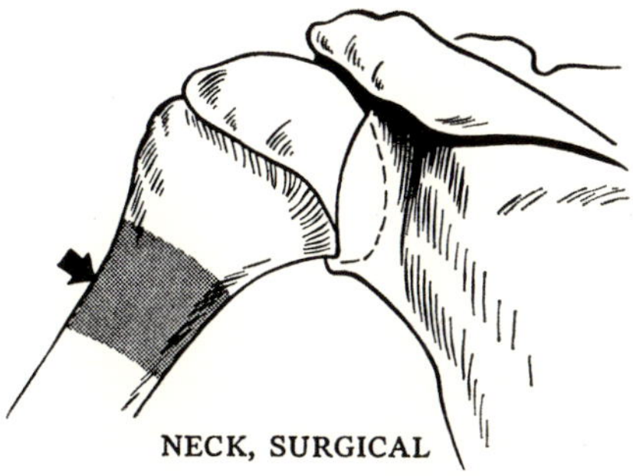

Figure 31. The surgical neck of the humerus, bone of the upper arm.

The Arm: The skeleton of the arm is composed of a single bone, the *humerus.* It extends from the glenoid cavity of the scapula to the elbow. The humerus consists of a shaft and two enlarged extremities. The rounded head of the upper end fits into the glenoid cavity of the scapula. Beneath the head are two bony processes, the *greater tubercle* and the *lesser tubercle.* Between the tubercles lies a groove, the *bicipital or intertubercular groove.* The region below the tubercles forms the *surgical neck* of the bone. The lower end of the humerus has two rounded processes. The one on the outer side is the *capitulum.* It forms a joint with the upper end of the radius, a bone of the forearm.

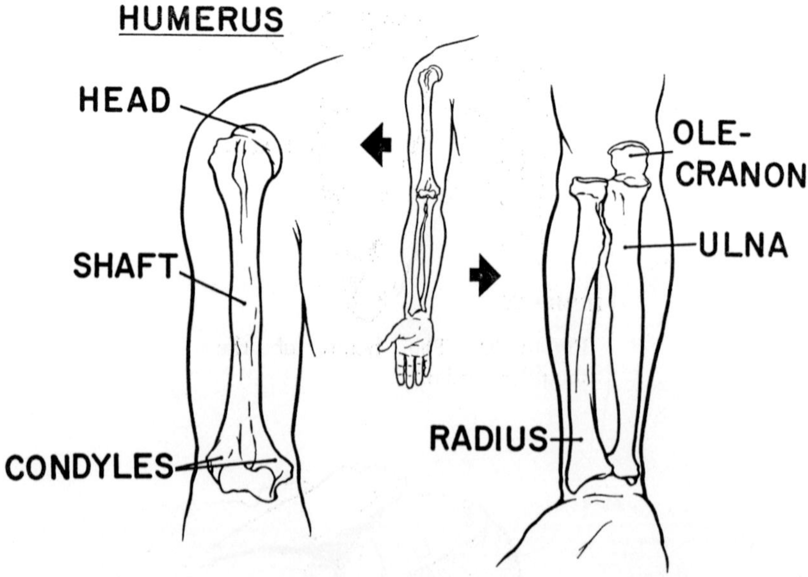

Figure 32. Bones of the arm: humerus, ulna, and radius.

The process on the inner side of the bone is the *trochlea.* It forms a joint with the upper end of the ulna, the other bone of the forearm. Just above the capitulum is a small bony projection, the *lateral epicondyle.* A similar projection, the *medial epicondyle,* is situated above the trochlea.

The Forearm: The bones of the forearm are the *ulna* and the *radius.* They extend from the elbow or lower end of the humerus to the wrist. The ulna is situated on the inner or medial side of the forearm, i.e. on the side of the little finger. At the upper end is the *olecranon,* a bony process forming the point of the elbow. Below the olecranon is a curved depression, the *semilunar notch,* which forms a joint with the trochlea of the humerus. Below the semilunar notch is a projection, the *coronoid process.* Near the coronoid process is a small groove, the *radial notch,* which forms a joint with the upper end of the radius. The lower end of the ulna is small and comprises a head (which is separated from the bones of the wrist by a piece of cartilage) and a sharp bony projection, the *styloid process.*

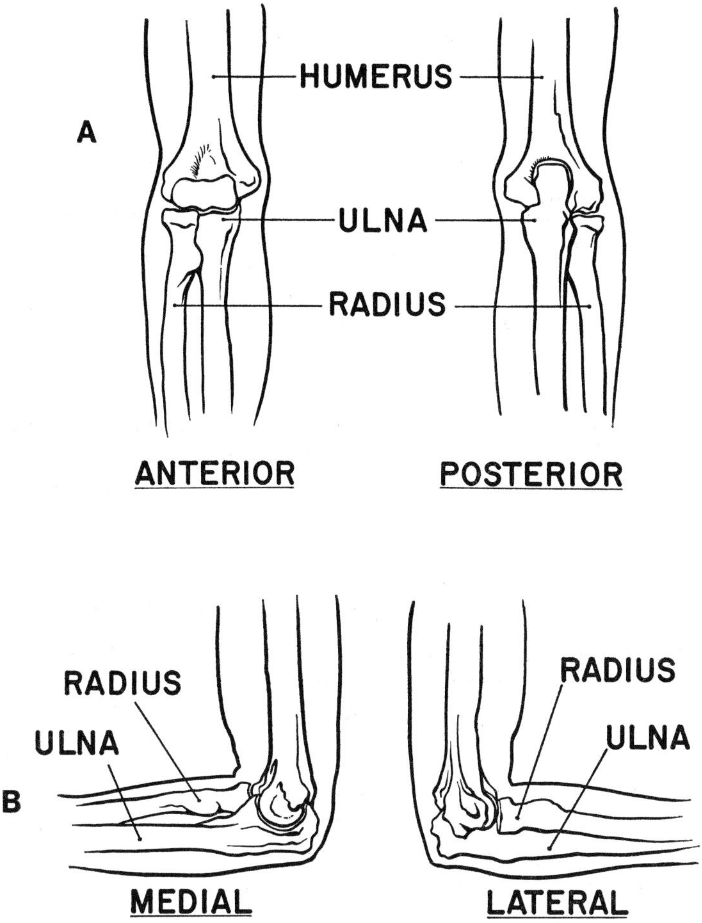

Figure 33. Four views of the bones of the elbow joint: *A*, Anterior and posterior. *B*, Medial and lateral.

The Radius: The outer bone of the forearm, the bone on the side of the thumb, is the radius. It is shorter than the ulna, but it is more massive below. The upper end has a disk-shaped head which forms a joint with the humerus and with the radial notch of the ulna. The massive lower end of the radius forms a joint with the bones of the wrist. It also has a styloid process similar to that of the ulna.

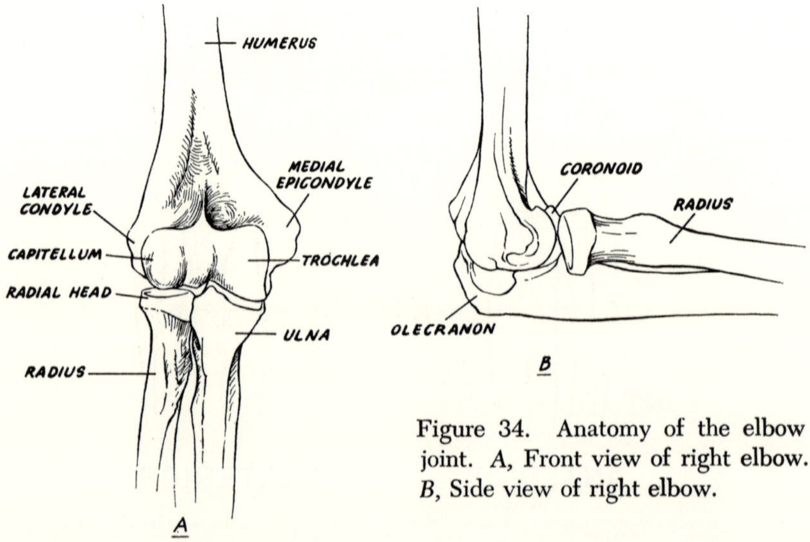

Figure 34. Anatomy of the elbow joint. *A*, Front view of right elbow. *B*, Side view of right elbow.

The Hand: The skeleton of the hand, including the wrist, is composed of 27 bones. The wrist is composed of eight small *carpal* bones. These are arranged in two rows, between the lower ends of the ulna and radius and the bones of the palm, the *metacarpal* bones. The metacarpal bones are five cylindrical bones extending through the palm between the wrist (or carpal bones) and the bones of the fingers. The skeleton of each finger, except the thumb, consists of three short cylindrical bones joined end to end. The thumb has only two bones. Each bone of a finger is known as a *phalanx* (plural *phalanges*).

THE LOWER EXTREMITY. The lower extremity consists of the thigh, the knee, the leg, the ankle, and the foot.

The Thigh: The *femur* or thigh bone is the longest and strongest bone of the body. Like the humerus, it consists of a shaft and two enlarged extremities. The upper end has a rounded head which forms a joint with the acetabulum of the innominate bone. The constricted portion below the head is the neck of the femur. This region is the common site of fractures in elderly persons. Below the neck are two bony processes, the *greater trochanter* and the *lesser trochanter*. The lower end of the femur

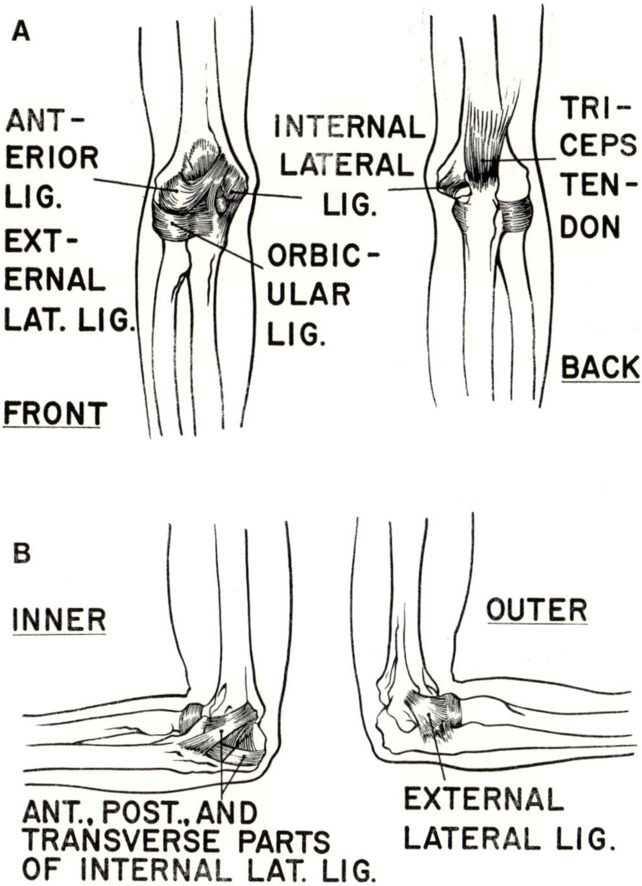

Figure 35. The important ligaments of the elbow joint. Diagram *A* shows anterior and posterior; *B* shows medial and lateral.

widens out into two bony eminences, the *lateral condyle* and the *medial condyle*.

The Knee: The bones of the knee comprise the lower end of the femur, the upper ends of the two bones of the leg, and the *patella* or kneecap. The patella is an oval bone situated in front of the knee joint. It is embedded in the tendon of the front thigh muscles, and it serves to protect the joint and to give the tendon more leverage in pulling on the leg.

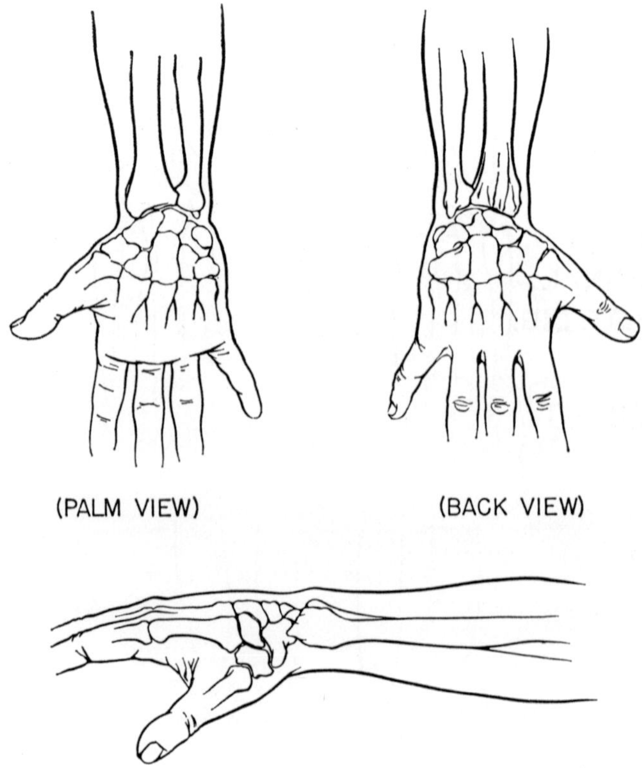

Figure 36. Three views of the bones of the wrist and forearm: palmar or volar, dorsal, and lateral.

The Leg: The skeleton of the leg consists of two bones, the *tibia* and the *fibula.* The tibia is the stouter or more massive bone, situated on the inner side of the leg (i.e. on the side of the big toe). The upper end, which forms a joint with the femur, is enlarged and shows two prominences, the *lateral condyle* and the *medial condyle.* In front of the bone, at the junction of the head and the shaft, is a bony prominence, the *tuberosity* of the tibia. At the lower end of the bone, on the inner side, there is a downward bony projection known as the *medial malleolus.* The other bone of the leg, the fibula, is situated parallel with the tibia on the outer side of the leg. The upper end of the fibula forms a joint with the upper end of the tibia, but it does not enter into

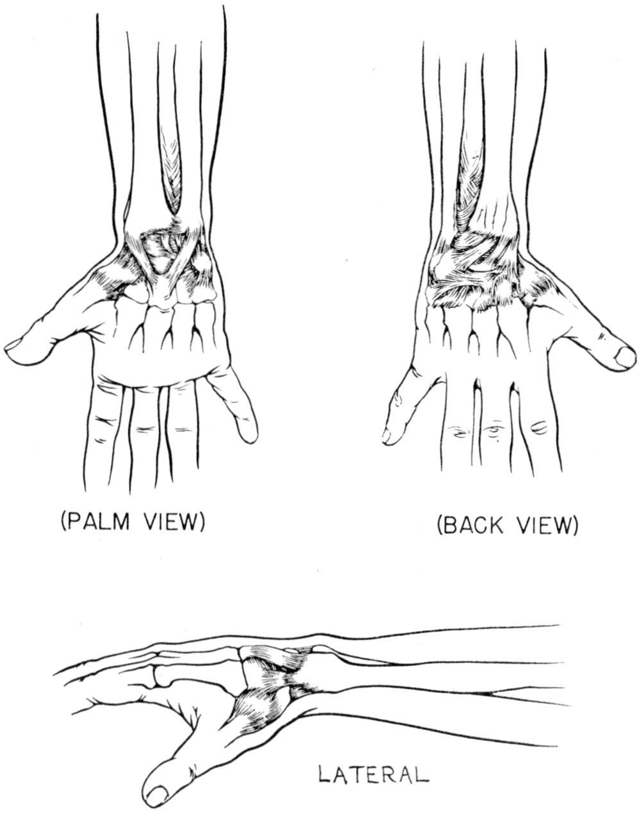

Figure 37. The ligaments of the wrist.

the formation of the knee joint. The lower end has a downward projection on its outer surface, the *lateral malleolus,* which together with the medial malleolus forms a joint at the ankle.

The Ankle: The ankle is the region between the leg and the foot where the lower ends of the tibia and fibula join the bones of the foot, especially the *talus,* the highest of the foot bones.

The Foot: The skeleton of the foot is composed of 26 bones. The back part of the foot comprises the seven *tarsal* bones, known collectively as the *tarsus.* The uppermost of the tarsal bones is the *talus,* which forms a joint with the lower ends of the tibia and the fibula. Below the talus is the *calcaneus* or heel bone. In

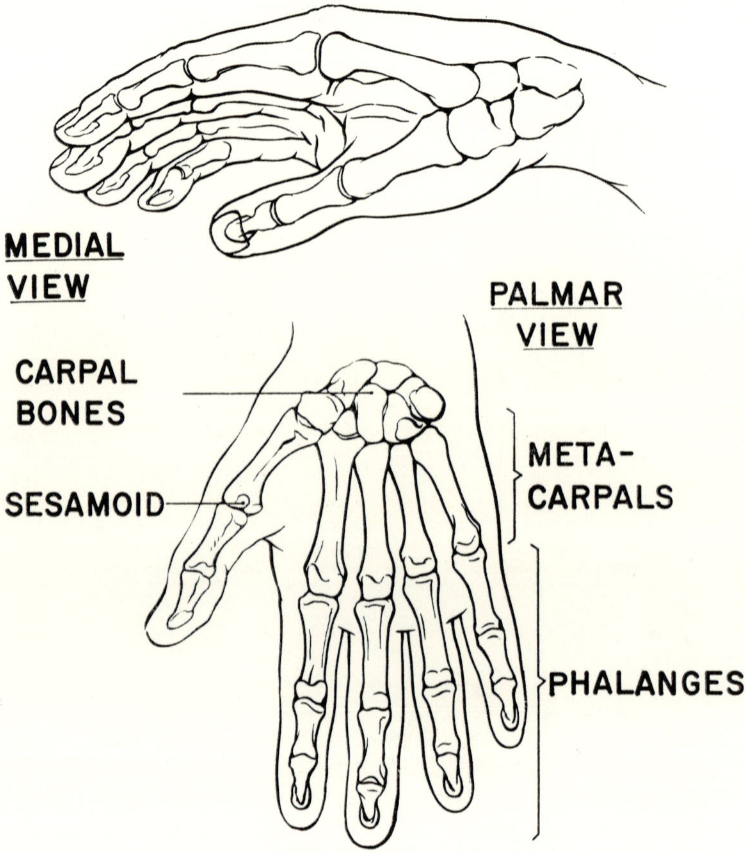

Figure 38. Bones of the hand: medial, and palmar or volar views.

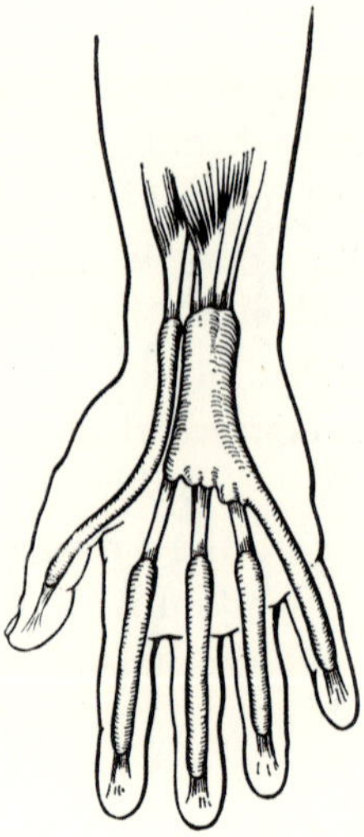

Figure 39. Palmar view of the tendon sheaths of the right hand.

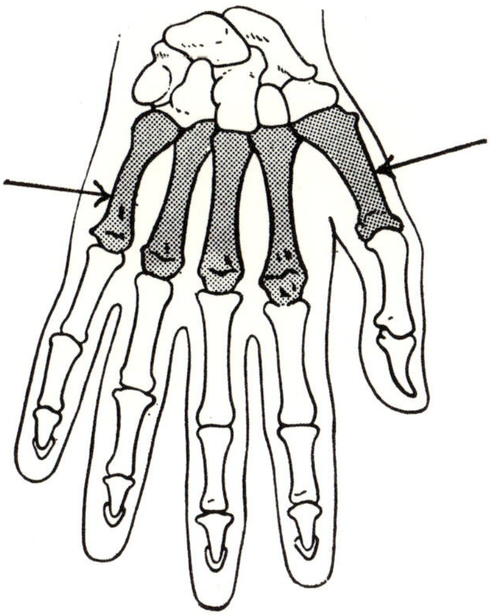

Figure 40. Metacarpal bones of hand.

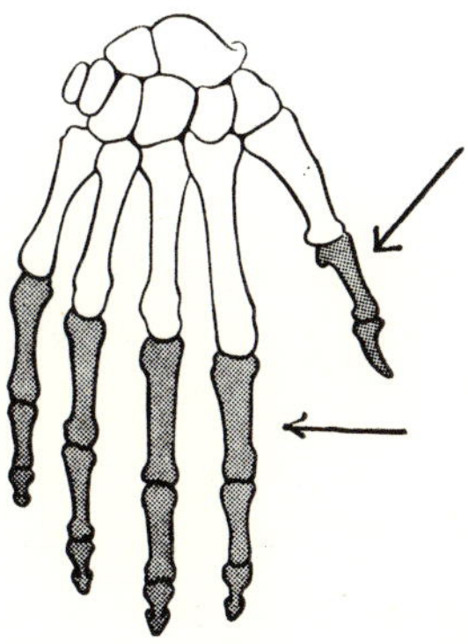

Figure 41. Phalanges of hand.

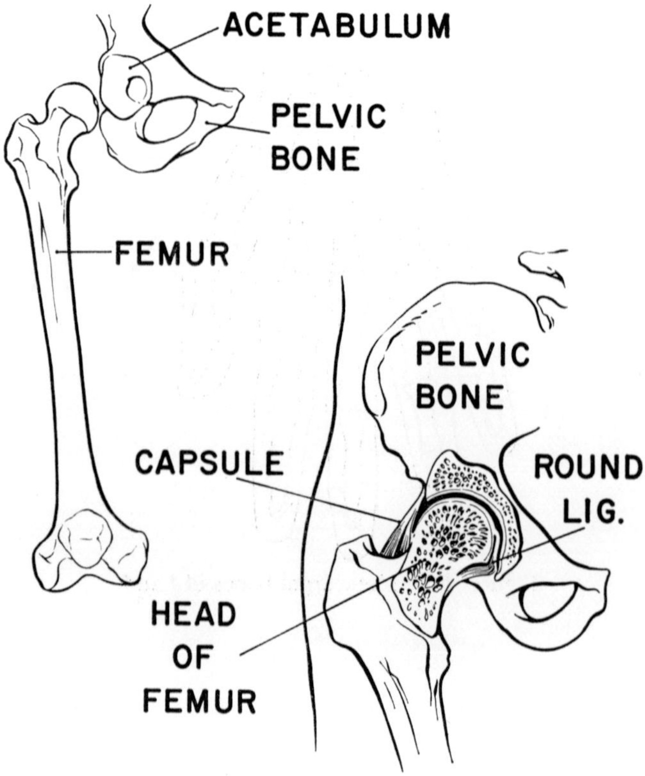

Figure 42. Cross-section of hip joint showing capsule and joint space.

front of the tarsal bones are the five *metatarsal* bones, which correspond to the metacarpal bones of the hand. The skeleton of the toes, like the skeleton of the fingers, is composed of three short cylindrical bones for each toe except the big toe, which has only two bones. Each such bone is known as a *phalanx* (plural *phalanges*).

VOCABULARY LESSON

On the basis of the preceding discussion, define the following terms. Determine the pronunciation with the aid of a medical dictionary.

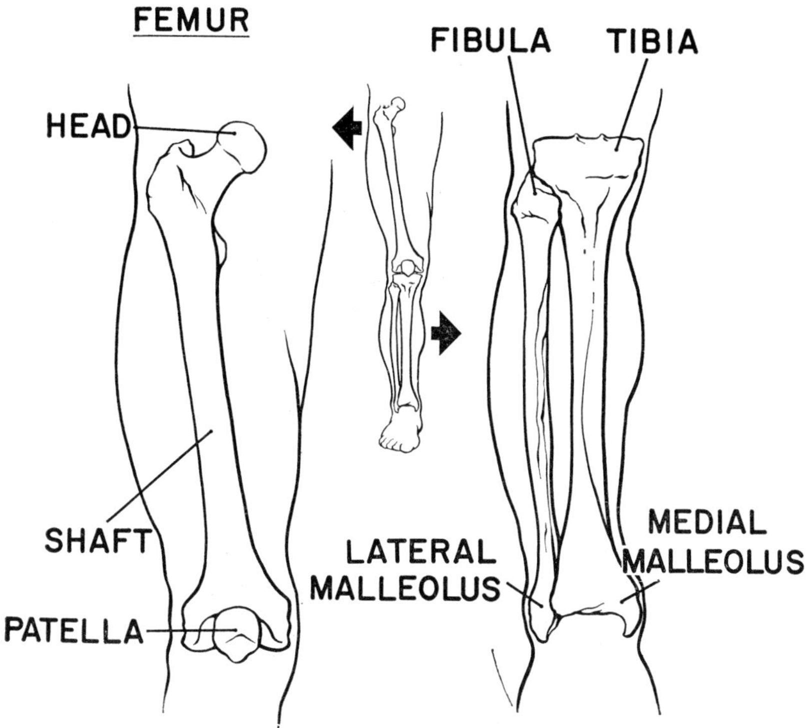

Figure 43. Diagram of bones of thigh and leg: femur, tibia (shinbone), fibula, and patella.

acetabulum
acromion process
atlas
axis
bicipital groove
calcaneus
capitulum
carpal bones
cervical
clavicle
coccyx
coracoid process
coronoid process
costal cartilage
ensiform
femur
fibula
gladiolus
glenoid cavity
greater trochanter
greater tubercle
humerus
ilium
inferior articular process
innominate bone
intertubercular groove
intervertebral disk
ischium
lamina
laminae
lateral condyle
lateral epicondyle
lesser trochanter
lesser tubercle
lumbar

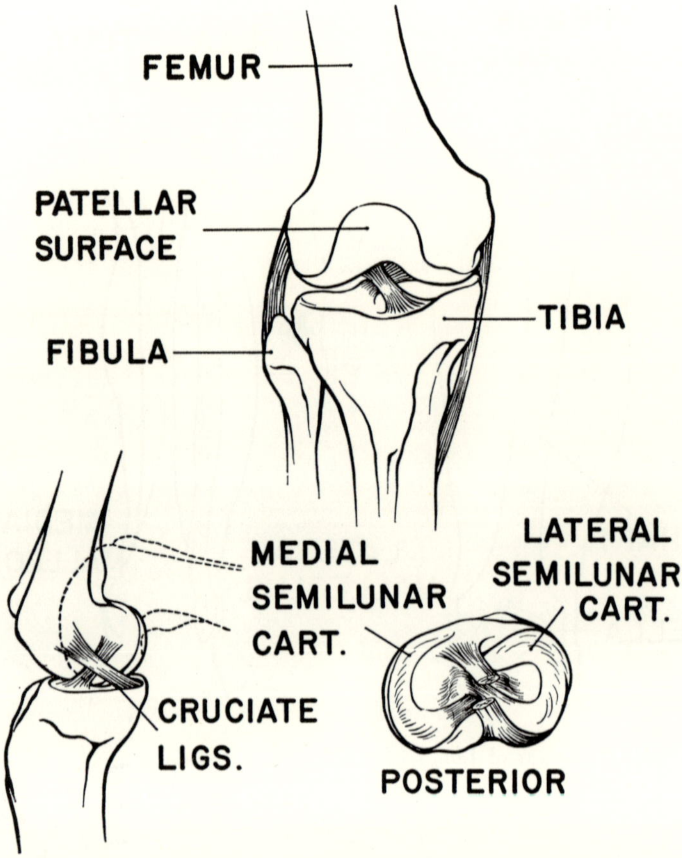

Figure 44. Bones and auxiliary structures of knee joint.

manubrium
medial condyle
medial epicondyle
medial malleolus
metacarpal bones
metatarsal bones
olecranon
patella
pedicle
pelvic cavity
pelvis
phalanges
phalanx
pubis
radial notch
radius
rib
sacral
sacrum
scapula
semilunar notch
shoulder girdle
spinal column
spinal cord
spine
spinous process
sternum
styloid process
superior articular process

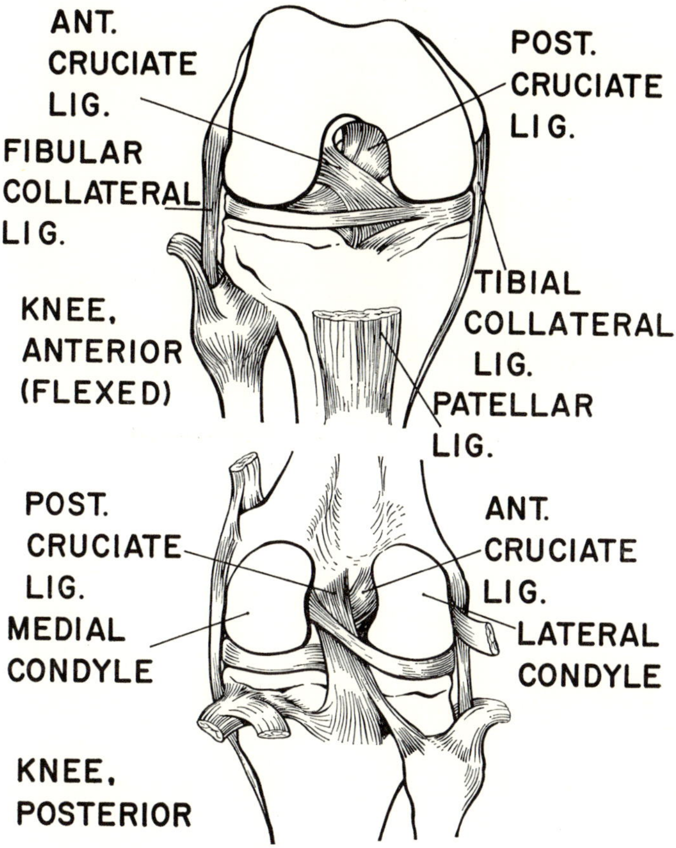

Figure 45. Anterior and posterior views of the knee joint showing the ligaments (lower diagram). Upper diagram shows knee in a flexed position.

surgical neck
symphysis pubis
talus
tarsal bones
tarsus
thoracic
thoracic vertebrae
thorax
tibia
transverse process
trochlea
tuberosity of tibia
ulna
vertebra
vertebrae
vertebral column
vertebral foramen
xiphoid

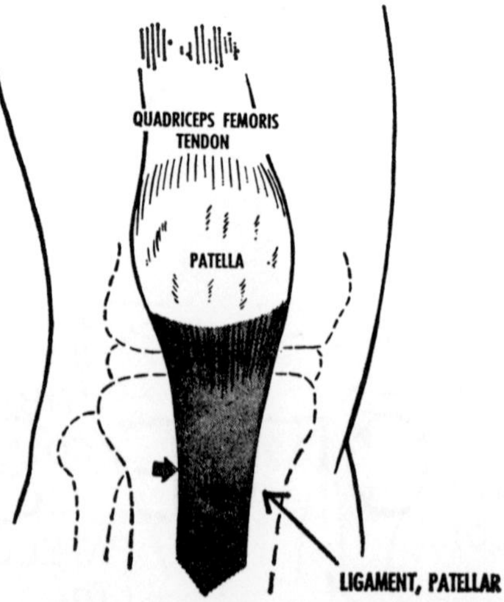

Figure 46. View of the patellar ligament, the patella, and the tendon of the quadriceps femoris, the muscles of the thigh which extend the leg at the knee.

VOCABULARY EXERCISE

Using a standard medical dictionary, determine the component parts of the following words:

bicipital	epicondyle
ensiform	metacarpal
innominate	metatarsal
intertubercular	semilunar
intervertebral	symphysis

What is the plural of the following words:

acetabulum	patella
axis	pelvis
capitulum	phalanx
coccyx	pubis
femur	radius
gladiolus	sacrum
humerus	scapula
ilium	talus
ischium	thorax
manubrium	vertebra

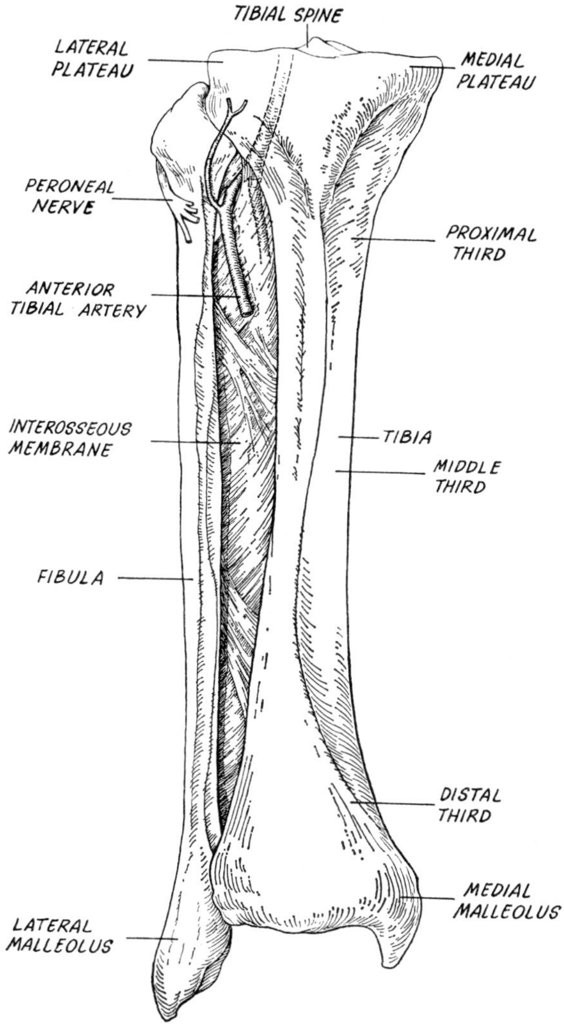

Figure 47. The bones of the leg: tibia and fibula. The tibia or shinbone is the more massive of the two bones, and it contributes more to the formation of the knee and ankle joints. Note the interosseous membrane, a heavy fibrous sheet, joining the two bones. It provides a place of origin for several of the muscles of the leg and foot.

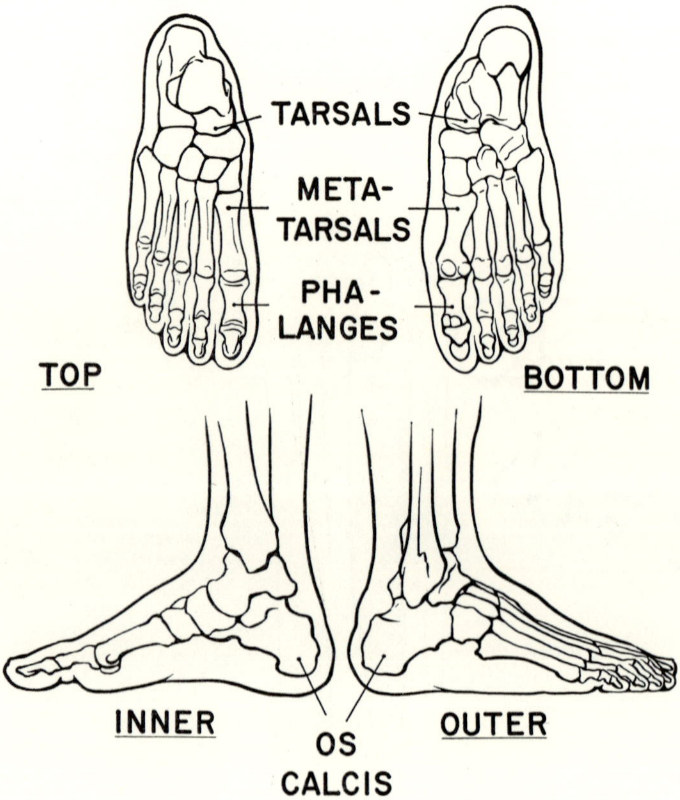

Figure 48. Four views of the bones of the foot: superior, inferior, medial, and lateral. The os calcis is the heel bone. The upper drawing shows the three groups of bones: the tarsals, the metatarsals, and the phalanges.

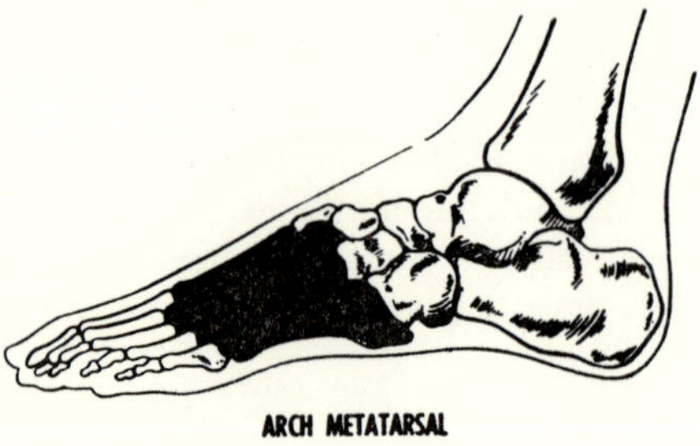

Figure 49. Side view of the metatarsal arch, the arch of the foot formed by the metatarsal bones.

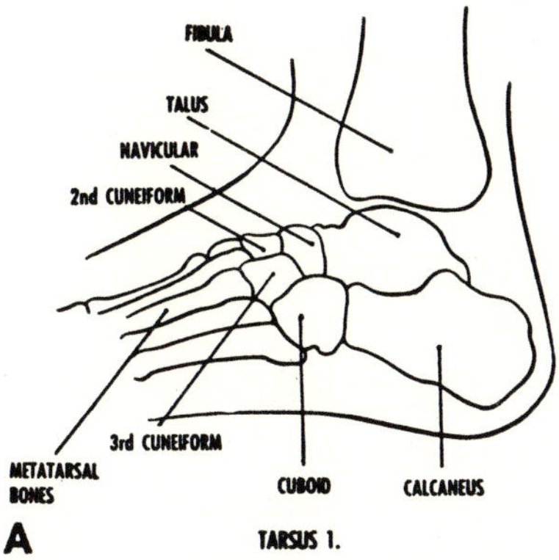

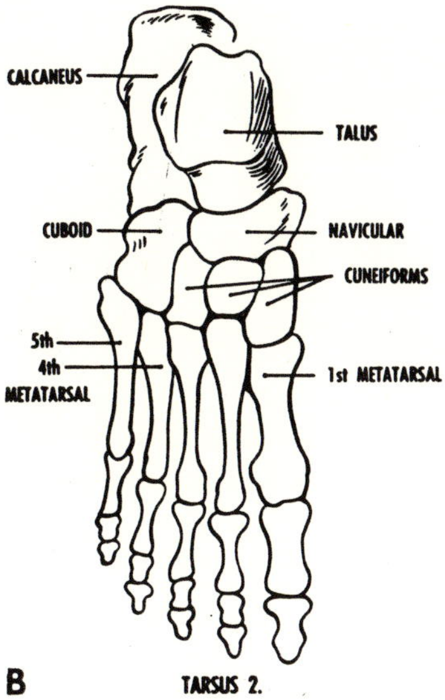

Figure 50. Bones of the tarsus and metatarsus. The tarsus is situated behind the metatarsal bones and is composed of seven bones: the calcaneus, talus, cuboid, navicular, and three cuneiforms.

Which of the words in the preceding chapter refer to the following concepts:

vinegar cruet	handle
little head	little hammer
cuckoo	chest
sword	pulley
little sword	elbow
shoulder	sacred

Give the medical term for the following structures:

first vertebra of neck	kneecap
heel bone	bones of fingers
collarbone	shoulder blade
bone of thigh	breastbone
hip bone	shinbone
bone of upper arm	bones of lower arm

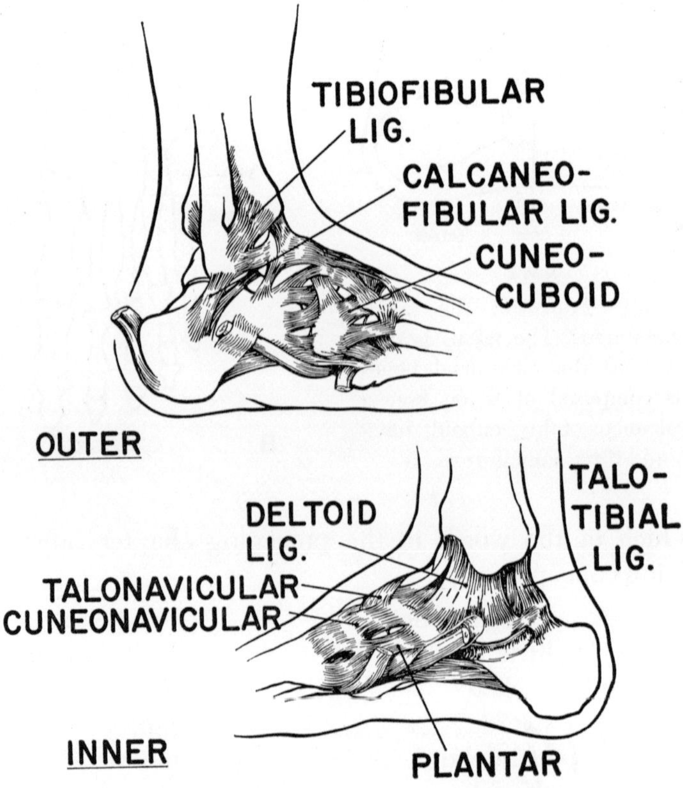

Figure 51. Medial and lateral views of the ligaments of the ankle and foot. Note calcaneofibular ligament on outer aspect of ankle and the deltoid ligament on inner aspect. These are occasionally torn in fractures of the ankle.

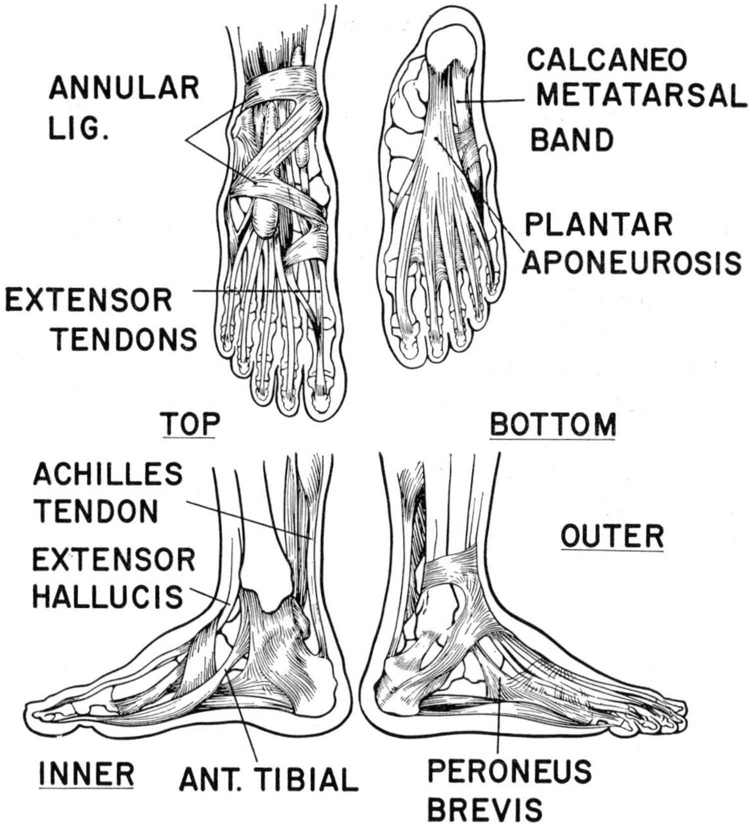

Figure 52. Tendons of the ankle and foot. Note annular ligament holding down the tendons.

Chapter V

BODY DIRECTIONS OR POSITIONS

A NUMBER OF TERMS are used in anatomy to designate positions or directions with reference to the body as a whole or to parts thereof. These terms help to locate the position of organs or other structures. In using these terms it is important to remember that they refer to the body in its so-called anatomical position, i.e. standing with the arms at the sides of the trunk and the palms turned forward.

Anterior or *ventral*: Designating the front part or surface of the body or a part thereof. The *kneecap* is on the *anterior* surface of the knee; the navel is on the *ventral* surface of the trunk.

Posterior or *dorsal*: Designating the back of the body, an organ, or a part thereof. The buttocks are on the *posterior* (or *dorsal*) aspect of the body.

Medial: Facing, or situated nearer, the midline of the body or the middle. The eye is *medial* to the ear (i.e. closer to the midline of the head than the ear is).

Lateral: Situated farther from the midline; toward the side. The eye is *lateral* to the nose.

Internal: Deep or deeper within the body. The *internal* carotid artery is deeper within the neck than the external carotid. The liver is an *internal* organ.

External: Near or nearer the surface of the body. The skin is the *external* covering of the body.

Superior: Situated above; in a higher position. The nose is *superior* to the mouth.

Inferior: Situated below; in a lower position. The mouth is *inferior* to the nose.

Proximal: Near or nearer to the body or to the point of attachment. The thigh is the *proximal* part of the lower limb.

Distal: Farther or farthest from the body or from the point of attachment. The segment of a finger bearing the nail is the *distal* part of the finger.

Central: Situated within or nearer the center of something. The brain and the spinal cord are described as the *central* nervous system, as opposed to the nerves of the limbs or skin.

Peripheral: Pertaining to, or directed toward, the exterior of the body. A nerve extending to the surface of the body is a *peripheral* nerve.

Cranial or *cephalic*: Nearer or nearest to the head; pertaining to the cranium. The *cranial* end of the spinal cord is the end near the brain.

Caudal: Close or closer to the lower part of the body; farther down. The *caudal* end of the spinal cord is situated in the lumbar vertebrae.

Parietal: Pertaining to the walls of the body or of a body cavity. The inner surface of the chest wall is lined by the *parietal* pleura.

Visceral: Pertaining to or involving an organ or organs. The surface of the lung is covered by the *visceral* pleura.

Afferent: Conducting or conveying *toward* a particular structure. Veins are *afferent* blood vessels carrying blood *toward* the heart. Sensory nerves are *afferent* nerves carrying impulses *toward* the brain or spinal cord.

Efferent: Conducting or conveying *away from* a particular structure. The arteries are *efferent* blood vessels carrying blood *away from* the heart. Motor nerves are *efferent* nerves conducting impulses *away from* the brain or spinal cord.

Sagittal: Designating an imaginary plane which divides the body into right and left portions.

Midsagittal: Designating an imaginary plane which divides the body into equal right and left portions; a vertical plane passing through the midline and dividing the body into two halves of equal size.

Frontal or *coronal*: Designating an imaginary vertical plane which divides the body into front and back portions; it is at right angles to a sagittal section or plane.

Transverse: Designating an imaginary plane in a horizontal direction (at right angles to both sagittal and frontal planes), which divides the body into upper and lower portions.

TERMS OF MOVEMENT

Flexion: A bending of a part on itself (as of the uterus) or a bending at a joint. The act of touching one's face with the hand involves *flexion* of the arm at the elbow.

Extension: The opposite of flexion; a straightening from a condition of flexion, as when the hand is moved away from the face or when the back is straightened from a slouching position.

Abduction: A movement away from the side or the midline of the body, as when the arm held at the side of the trunk is moved away and upward.

Adduction: The opposite of abduction; a movement, as of the arm, toward the side of the body.

Circumduction: The complex movement involved when a circle is drawn, as on a board, with the arm outstretched. Drawing a circle with the toe, as in the sand, involves circumduction of the lower limb.

Rotation: The turning of a part, as the arm, head, or trunk, on its axis, as when the head is turned to the side.

Pronation: A kind of rotatory movement of an upper or lower limb. In the case of the arm, *pronation* is the movement involved when the hand unscrews the lid of jar. For the left arm, *pronation* is involved when the lid of a jar is screwed on.

Supination: A rotatory movement which is the opposite of *pronation*. The unscrewing of a jar lid with the left hand involves *supination*.

Inversion: The movement of the foot which makes the sole face the opposite foot; a movement at the ankle joint which turns the foot in such a way that its sole faces the midline of the body.

Eversion: A movement which is opposite to inversion; a movement of a foot which makes the sole face outward.

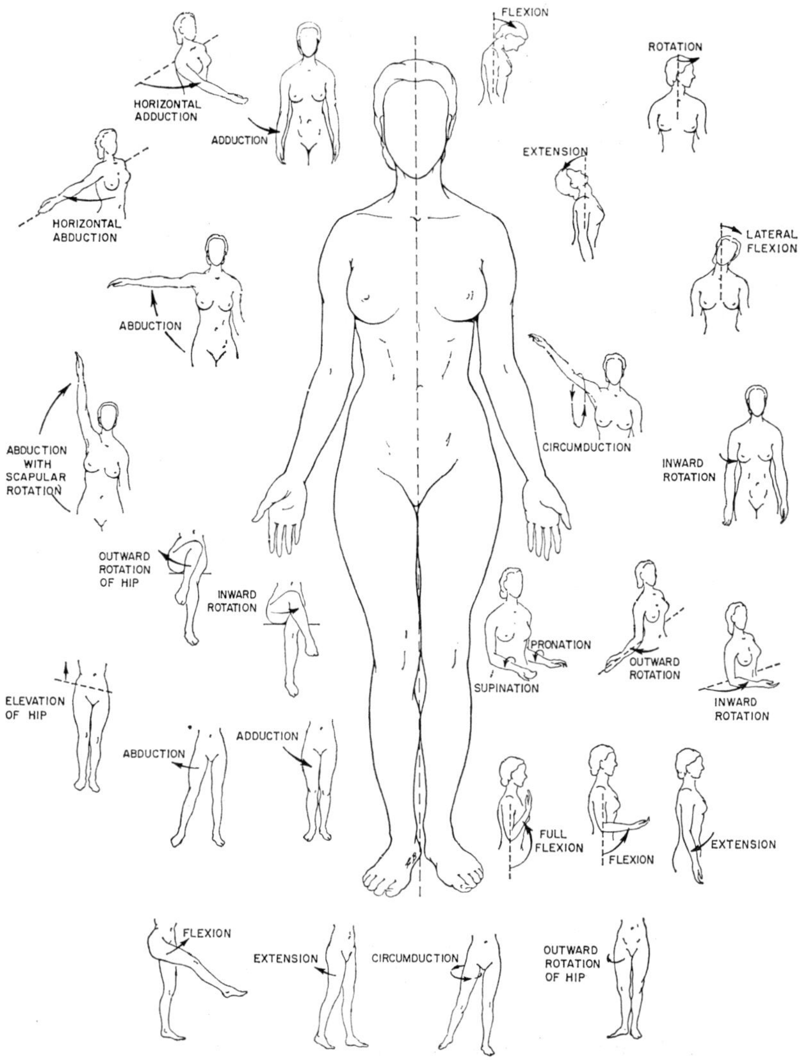

Figure 53. Terms used in anatomy to designate movement or position.

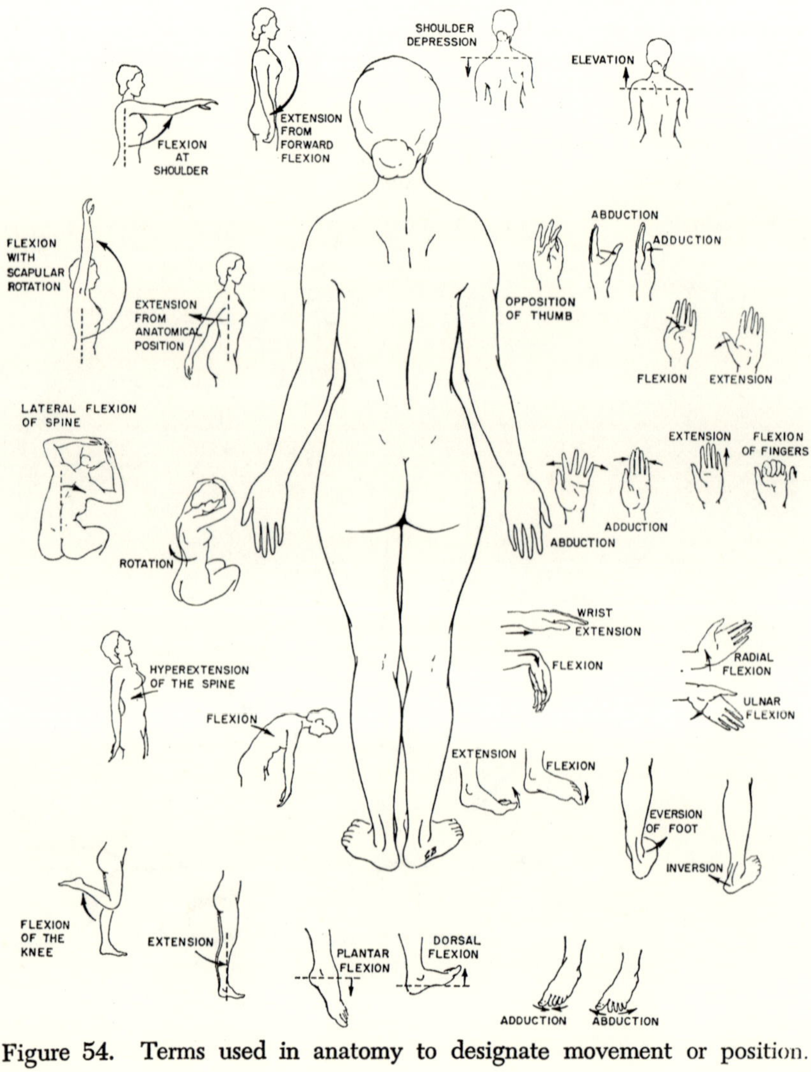

Figure 54. Terms used in anatomy to designate movement or position.

VOCABULARY REVIEW

On the basis of the preceding lesson, define the following terms. Determine the pronunciation by consulting a medical dictionary.

abduction	efferent	parietal
adduction	eversion	peripheral
afferent	extension	posterior
anterior	external	pronation
caudal	flexion	proximal
central	frontal	rotation
cephalic	inferior	sagittal
circumduction	internal	superior
coronal	inversion	supination
cranial	lateral	transverse
distal	medial	ventral
dorsal	midsagittal	visceral

VOCABULARY EXERCISE

With the aid of a medical dictionary, show the combining forms from which the following terms are compounded:

abduction	inversion
adduction	midsagittal
afferent	peripheral
circumduction	

What words have the opposite meaning of the following terms?

abduction	dorsal
afferent	eversion
anterior	extension
caudal	external
central	inferior
distal	lateral

Chapter VI

THE MUSCULAR SYSTEM

THE FUNCTION OF MUSCLES. Movements of parts of the body with reference to one another, as well as movement of the body as a whole, is accomplished by one or more muscles or by groups of muscles. A typical muscle may be envisioned as having the shape of an Indian club, thick in the center and tapering toward the ends. The thick portion of the muscle is the *belly*. The thinner ends, consisting of tough fibrous tissue, are called *tendons*. To induce movement, a muscle contracts, thereby shortening the distance between its ends while becoming thicker in the middle.

ATTACHMENT OF MUSCLES. With a few exceptions, the two ends of a muscle are attached to different bones having one or more joints between them. Generally, one end, known as the *origin*, is attached to a nonmoving or less-movable bone. The other end, the *insertion*, is attached to the bone or other part which the muscle is intended to move. When the muscle contracts it becomes shorter, and since one end (the origin) is relatively immovable, the other end (the insertion) must perforce move and carry the bone with it. A typical example of this is found in the biceps muscle of the arm. The origin of the biceps is attached to the relatively stable scapula, while the insertion is attached to the bones of the forearm. When the biceps contracts, the arm is bent at the elbow and the forearm is carried toward the shoulder.

STRUCTURE OF MUSCULAR TISSUE. Muscular tissue or a muscle is composed of fine elastic threads that may be envisioned as strands of hair. Each thread is a muscle *fiber*. Each fiber is actually an elongated cell. Muscle fibers are arranged in bundles. Each bundle of muscle fibers is known as a *fasciculus* (plural *fasciculi*). Several fasciculi form a muscle. The entire muscle is surrounded by a sheath of connective tissue called *fascia.*

TYPES OF MUSCLES. There are three types of muscle tissue: *striated, smooth,* and *cardiac.* Striated muscle is so called because it gives the appearance, under the microscope, of being striped. Striated muscles are under the control of the will and are therefore also called *voluntary* muscles. They are also known as *skeletal* muscles because they are attached to the bones of the skeleton. Smooth muscle, also known as *involuntary* muscle and *visceral muscle,* is not under the control of the will. Such muscle tissue is found in the digestive organs (as the walls of the stomach and intestine), in the blood vessels, and other structures. Cardiac muscle is found in the walls of the heart. Under the microscope it is seen to have stripes, but unlike skeletal muscle it is not under the control of the will. It works automatically.

MUSCLE TONE. Normal muscles are in a state of slight tension even when they are relaxed or not in action. This condition keeps the muscles in shape and ready to function. *Muscle tone* is also known as *tonus* and *tonicity.*

SOME IMPORTANT MUSCLES

NECK AND SHOULDER. The *sternocleidomastoid* muscle (one on each side of the neck) is a strong muscle which helps in holding the head erect. When it is injured, as in childbirth, the head becomes abnormally drawn to one side or the other, depending on the condition of the muscle. The condition is known as *torticollis* or *wryneck.* The *deltoid* muscle covers the shoulder and the upper part of the arm. It is used as a site for *intramuscular* injection (injection into the substance of a muscle). Three other muscles situated in the back of the neck and head assist in rotating, inclining, and extending the head. They are the *splenius capitis, semispinalis capitis,* and *longissimus capitis.*

ARM AND ANTERIOR CHEST. The *biceps* muscle, located on the front of the upper arm, functions to flex or bend the arm at the elbow. The *triceps* muscle, situated on the back of the upper arm, extends or straightens the arm at the elbow. The *pectoralis major, pectoralis minor,* and the *serratus anterior* are strong

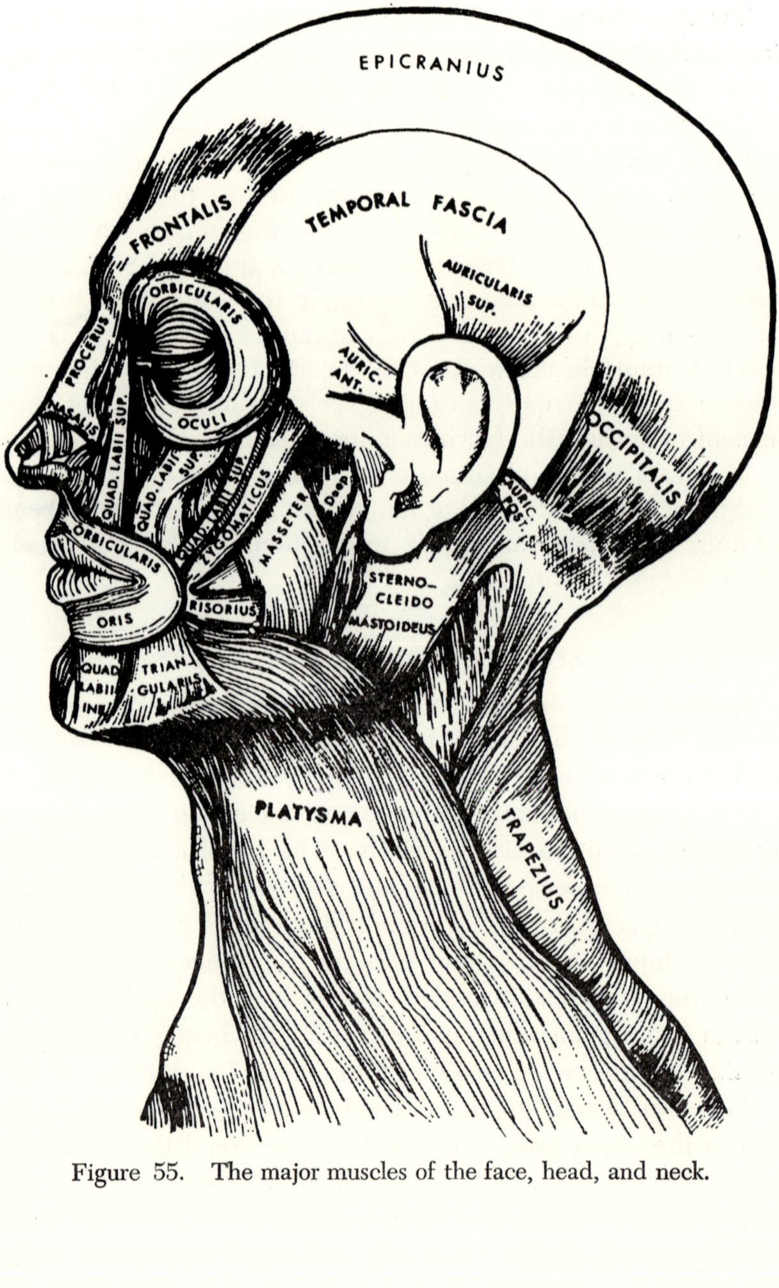

Figure 55. The major muscles of the face, head, and neck.

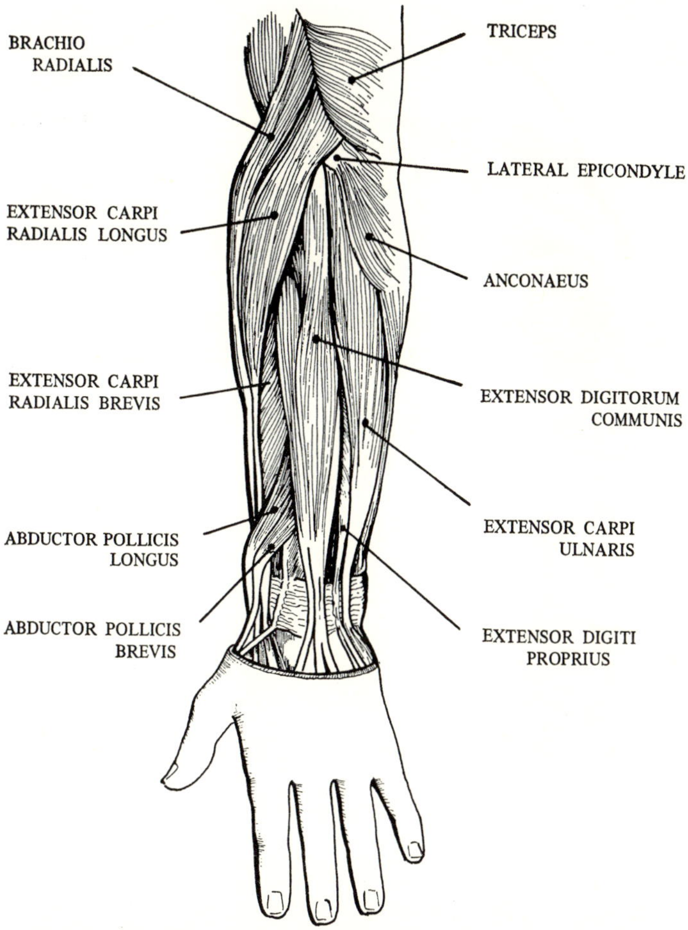

Figure 56. Muscles of the forearm as seen from the back.

muscles situated on the front part of the chest. The pectoralis major adducts and rotates the arm.

THE ABDOMEN. The muscles of the abdominal wall in front and the sides consist mainly of flat bands or sheets extending from the ribs to the pelvis or hips. They are the *internal oblique, external oblique, transversus abdominis,* and the *rectus abdominis.* Certain regions of the abdominal wall, especially where blood vessels or other structures pass through it, are rather weak and

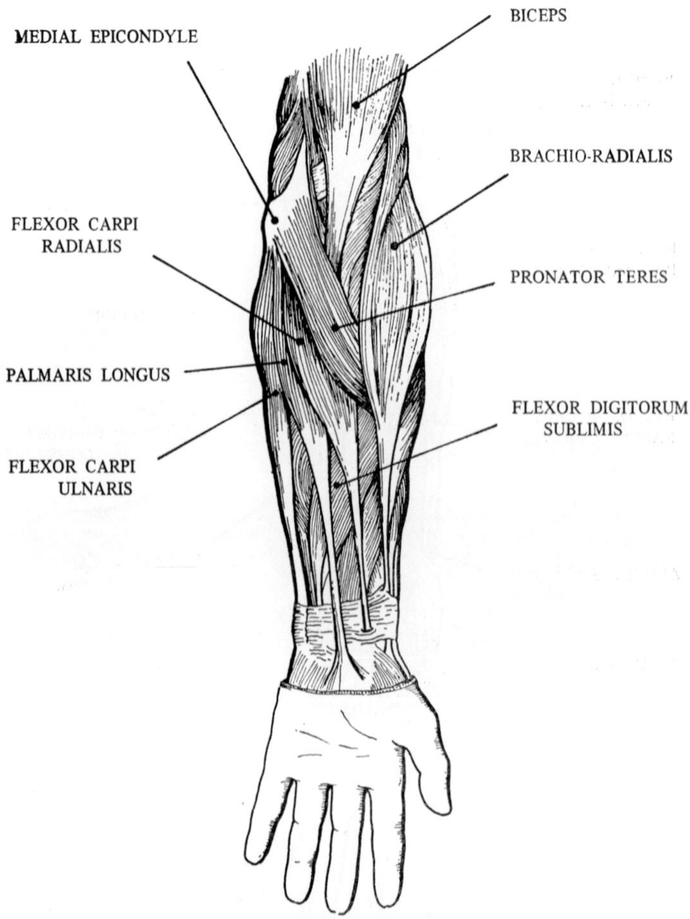

Figure 57. Muscles of the forearm as seen from the front.

often become the sites of a rupture or *hernia*. The *inguinal rings* (one on each side), the *femoral rings*, and the navel or *umbilicus* are common hernial sites. When a hernia occurs, some structure contained in the abdomen (such as a piece of intestine) protrudes through the weakened spot.

THE BACK. The two large muscles of the back are the *trapezius* (upper part of back) and the *latissimus dorsi* (below the trapezius). The trapezius moves the shoulder blade and the shoulder region.

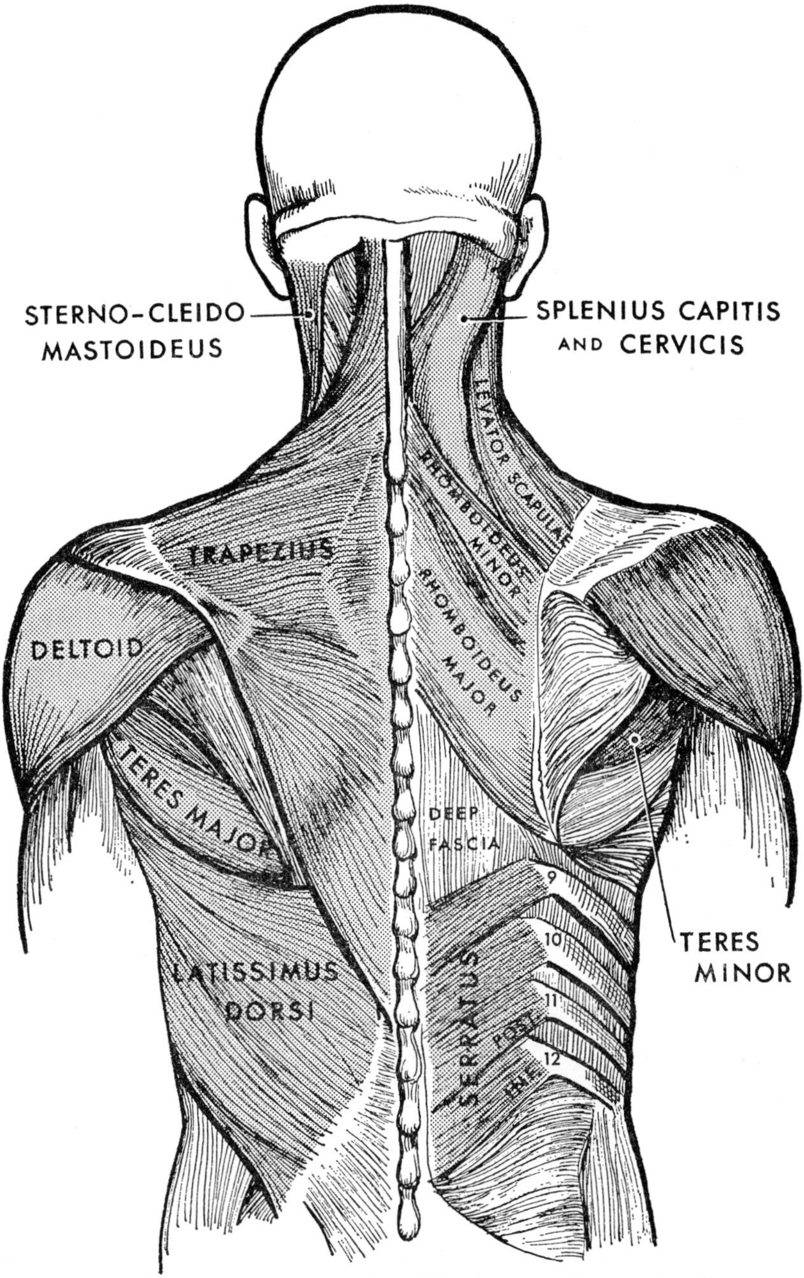

Figure 58. The major muscles of the back, neck, and shoulders.

The latissimus dorsi is concerned mainly with the movement of the upper arm.

THE BUTTOCKS. Each buttock is formed mainly by the *gluteus maximus* (the outer or superficial of the three muscles), the *gluteus medius* (under the gluteus maximus), and the *gluteus minimus* (under the gluteus medius). The three muscles are used in walking and in arising from a sitting position. The buttock is a site for intramuscular injections.

THIGH AND LEG. The following four muscles, situated in the front of the thigh, extend the leg at the knee: the *rectus femoris, vastus lateralis, vastus medialis,* and *vastus intermedius.* As a group they are known as the *quadriceps femoris.* The *hamstring* muscles on the back of the thigh are the *semitendinosus, semimembranosus,* and *biceps femoris.* They flex or bend the leg at the knee. The *sartorius,* the longest muscle of the body, passes obliquely across the front of the thigh. It flexes the leg. The *gracilis,* on the inner side of the thigh, adducts the thigh and flexes the leg. The *tibialis anterior,* on the front of the leg, flexes the foot and turns it inward. The *gastrocnemius* muscle, the *soleus,* and the *peroneus longus* give the calf its rounded appearance. All three extend the foot. The tendon which attaches the gastrocnemius and soleus muscles to the *calcaneus,* the bone of the heel, is known as *Achilles tendon.* It occasionally tears under excessive strain.

MUSCLES OF RESPIRATION. The most important muscle of breathing is the *diaphragm,* a dome-shaped sheet of muscle tissue situated horizontally within the body, between the chest and the abdomen. When the diaphragm contracts, its central portion moves downward, toward the abdomen, thus increasing the capacity of the chest and creating a partial vacuum around the lungs, causing air to flow into the lungs. When the diaphragm relaxes, its dome-shaped center moves upward and exerts pressure on the lungs, thus causing the air to flow out. The *intercostal* muscles, situated between the ribs, also help in respiration by alternately enlarging and decreasing the capacity of the chest cavity.

VOCABULARY REVIEW

Define the following terms on the basis of the preceding lesson. Consult a medical dictionary for the pronunciation.

Achilles tendon
belly
biceps
biceps femoris
calcaneus
cardiac
diaphragm
fascia
fasciculus
femoral rings
fiber
gastrocnemius
gluteus maximus
gluteus medius
gluteus minimus
gracilis
hamstring
hernia
inguinal rings
insertion
intercostal
internal oblique
intramuscular
involuntary
latissimus dorsi
longissimus capitis
muscle tone
origin
pectoralis major
pectoralis minor
peroneus longus
quadricept femoris
sartorius
serratus anterior
semimembranosus
semispinalis capitis
semitendinosus
skeletal
smooth muscle
soleus
splenius capitis
sternocleidomastoid
striated muscle
rectus abdominis
rectus femoris
tendon
tibialis anterior
tonicity
tonus
torticollis
transversus abdominis
trapezius
triceps
umbilicus
vastus intermedius
vastus lateralis
vastus medialis
visceral
voluntary muscle
wryneck

REVIEW QUESTIONS

1. What is the *belly* of a muscle?
2. What term describes the *tough fibrous tissue at the end of a muscle?*
3. What is the difference between the *origin* and the *insertion* of a muscle?
4. What term describes a bundle of muscle fibers?
5. What are the three types of muscle?
6. What is the name of the large muscle on each side of the neck?
7. What muscle covers the shoulder?

8. What muscle is situated on the front of the upper arm?
9. What muscle is in the back of the upper arm?
10. What are the two main muscles situated on the front of the chest?
11. Where is the *internal oblique muscle* located?
12. What are the three common hernial sites?
13. What are the two large muscles of the back?
14. What muscles form the bulk of the buttock?
15. What four muscles of the thigh are known as the *quadriceps femoris?*
16. What muscles are known as the *hamstring muscles*?
17. What muscles give the calf of the leg its rounded appearance?
18. What is the *Achilles tendon?*

Chapter VII

THE CIRCULATORY SYSTEM

COMPONENT PARTS. The circulatory system comprises the blood and the various organs and structures concerned with the circulation of the blood through the body. The blood consists of a fluid portion, the *plasma*, and the formed elements consisting of red blood cells or *erythrocytes*, white blood cells or *leukocytes*, and *platelets* or *thrombocytes*. The chief organ of the system is

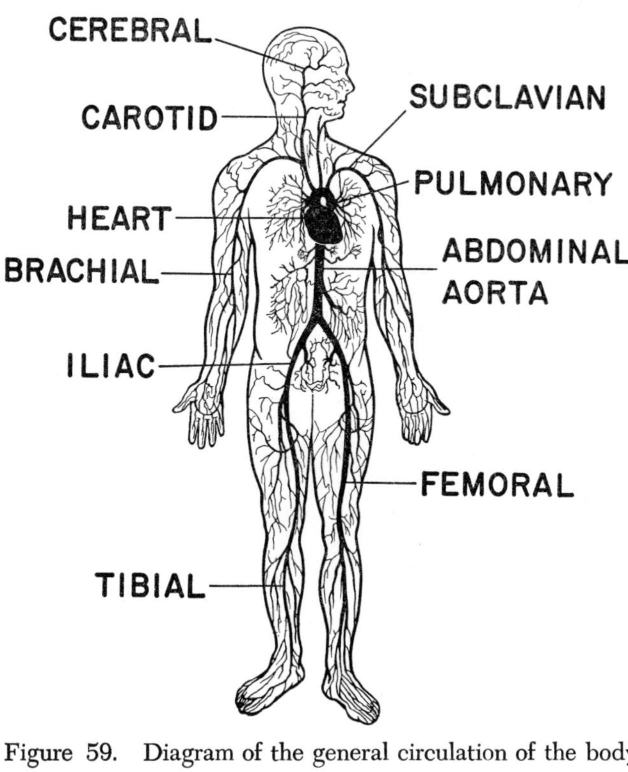

Figure 59. Diagram of the general circulation of the body.

the heart, which acts in the manner of a pump. The other structures are the *blood vessels,* by which the blood is conveyed to the various parts of the body. The chief blood vessels are the *arteries,* the *veins,* and the *capillaries.* The arteries, which vary in size, carry the blood from the heart toward the tissues or organs. The veins carry the blood from tissues or organs back to the heart. The capillaries are the finest blood vessels which connect the smaller arteries with the network of veins. The heart and the blood vessels form a closed and continuous system some-

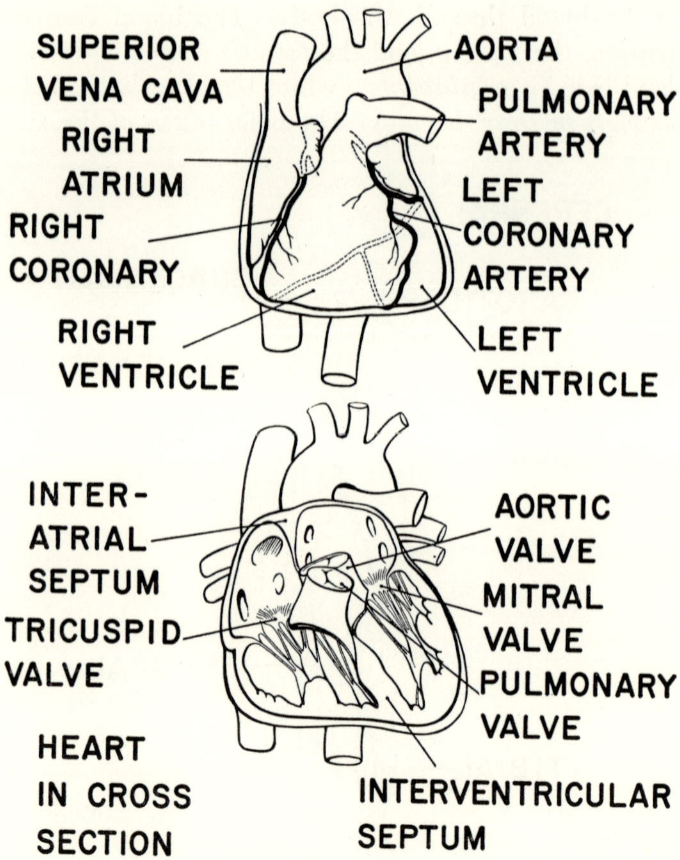

Figure 60. The upper diagram shows the front aspect of the heart and the relation of the large blood vessels to the chambers of the heart. The lower diagram shows the heart in cross-section.

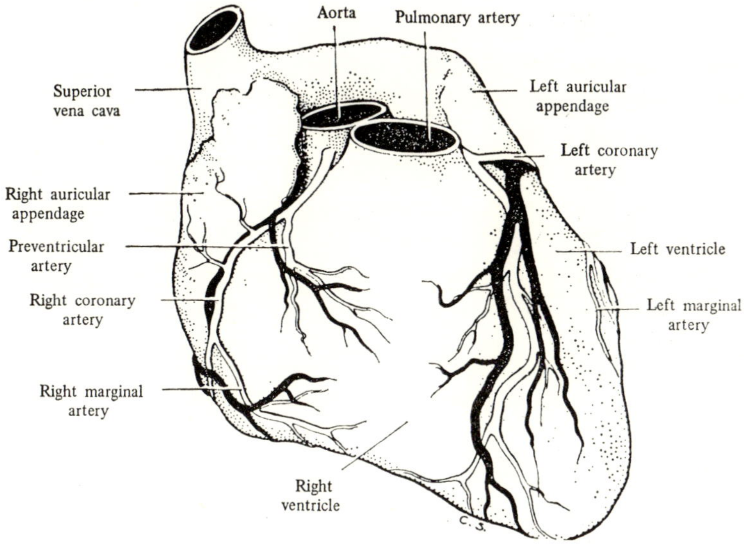

Figure 61. Arteries supplying blood to the muscular walls of the heart.

what analogous to the cooling system of an automobile. The heart is comparable to the water pump.

FUNCTIONS OF THE CIRCULATORY SYSTEM. The function of the heart is to circulate the blood through the network of arteries, capillaries, and veins, so that the blood may reach the tissues and cells of the body. The function of the blood is to carry oxygen to the cells and waste products, such as carbon dioxide, from the cells. The blood also carries food, hormones, and other substances.

STRUCTURE OF BLOOD CELLS. Under the microscope a red blood cell appears as a pink disk, somewhat thinner in the center than at the edges. The color is imparted by the presence of the pigment *hemoglobin,* the substance which enables the blood to carry oxygen. A normal red blood cell contains no nucleus. The leukocytes are of two principal kinds, the *granular* (which contain small granules) and the *nongranular.* The granular leukocytes are further subdivided into *basophils* (which stain readily with basic or alkaline dyes), *eosinophils* (which stain with acid dyes), and *neutrophils.*

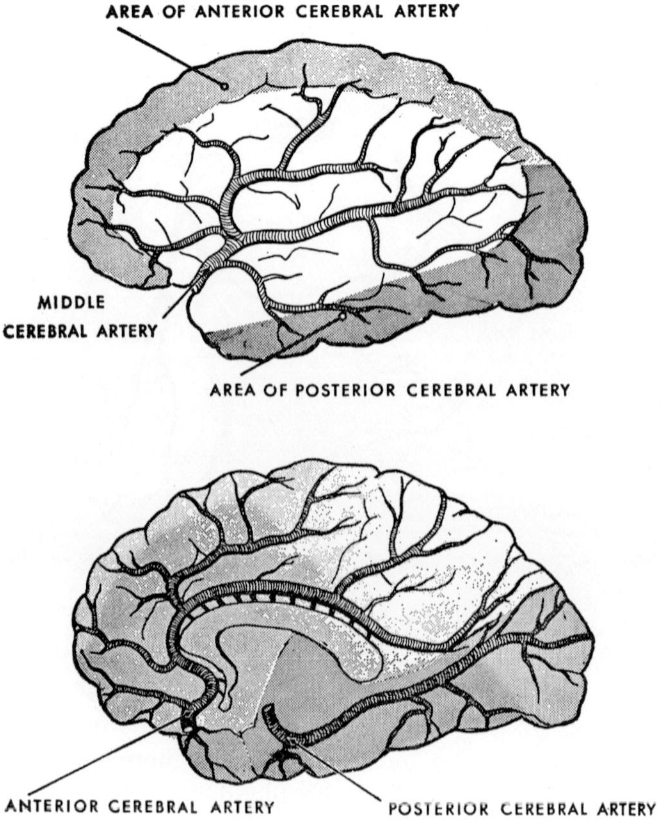

Figure 62. Vital arteries of the brain. Schematic shows lateral surface (upper illustration) and medial surface (lower illustration) of cerebrum and the regions supplied by the three cerebral arteries.

The nongranular leukocytes are divided into two subgroups, the *lymphocytes* and the *monocytes*. An increase in the number of leukocytes in the blood stream, as may occur in case of an infection, is known as *leukocytosis*. The blood platelets are smaller than the erythrocytes and leukocytes. They assist in the clotting or *coagulation* of blood.

STRUCTURE OF THE HEART. The heart is essentially a sack having thick muscular walls capable of contracting and relaxing. The inner surface of the heart is lined with a membrane known as *endocardium*. The outer surface is covered by another

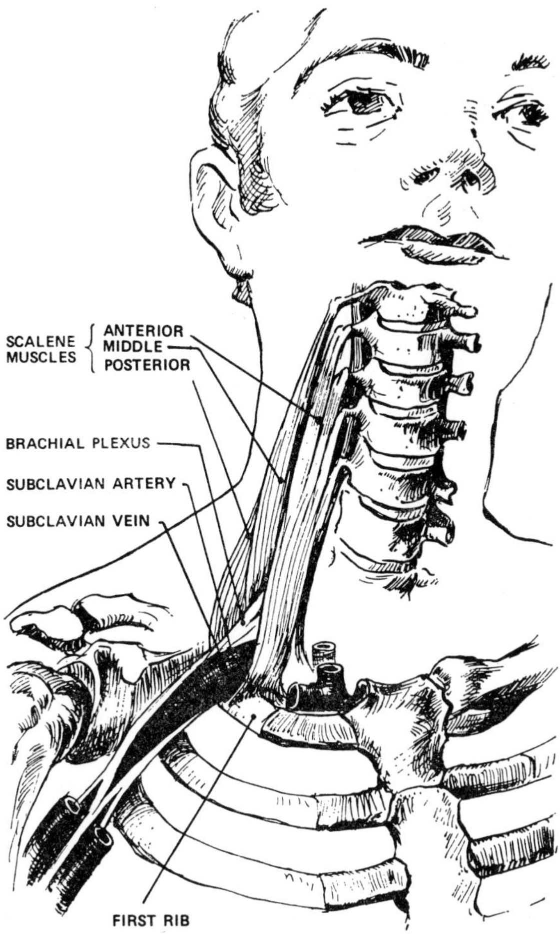

Figure 63. The large blood vessels of the neck in relation to the neck muscles and the brachial nerve plexus.

membrane called *pericardium*. The interior or cavity of the heart is divided into four chambers. First, a vertical partition divides the interior into right and left halves. The right half is concerned with the blood returned through the veins. The left side propels the blood into the arteries. Each side is further divided by a horizontal partition into an upper chamber and a lower chamber. The upper chamber is known as an *atrium* or *auricle;* the lower chamber, as a *ventricle*. The upper and lower chambers (i.e. the

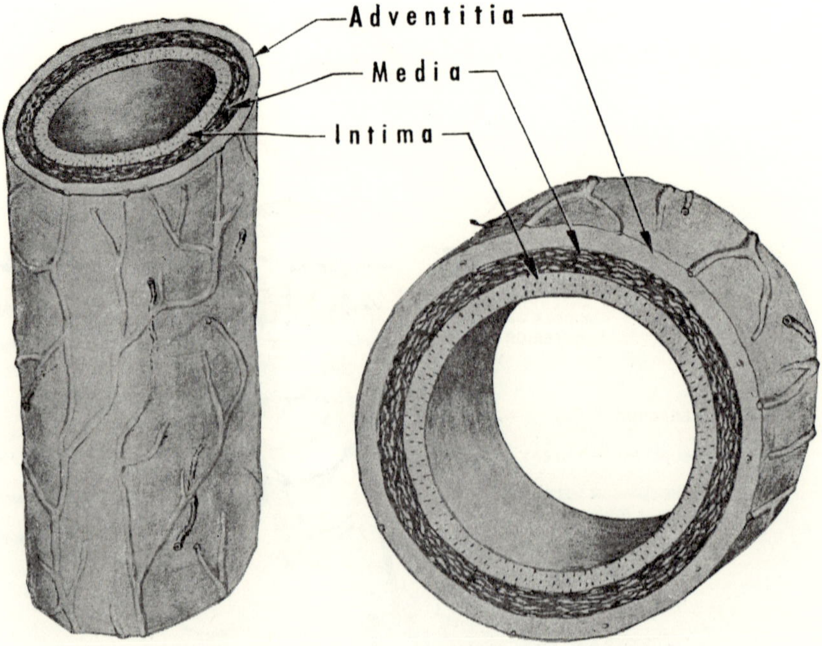

Figure 64. Cross-sections of an artery showing the three coats: adventitia, media, and intima.

atrium and the ventricle) communicate through an opening which is controlled by a valve that allows the blood to flow only in one direction, from the atrium to the ventricle. The valve between the right atrium and the right ventricle is called the *tricuspid valve.* The corresponding valve on the left side is called the *bicuspid* or *mitral valve.* The blood returning to the heart through the veins enters the right atrium and is propelled into the right ventricle. Contraction of the right ventricle forces the blood into the lungs, where it receives a fresh supply of oxygen. The oxygenated or refreshed blood then enters the left atrium and from there into the left ventricle. The contraction of the left ventricle forces the blood into the *aorta,* the large artery at the outlet of the ventricle. From the aorta, the blood is distributed

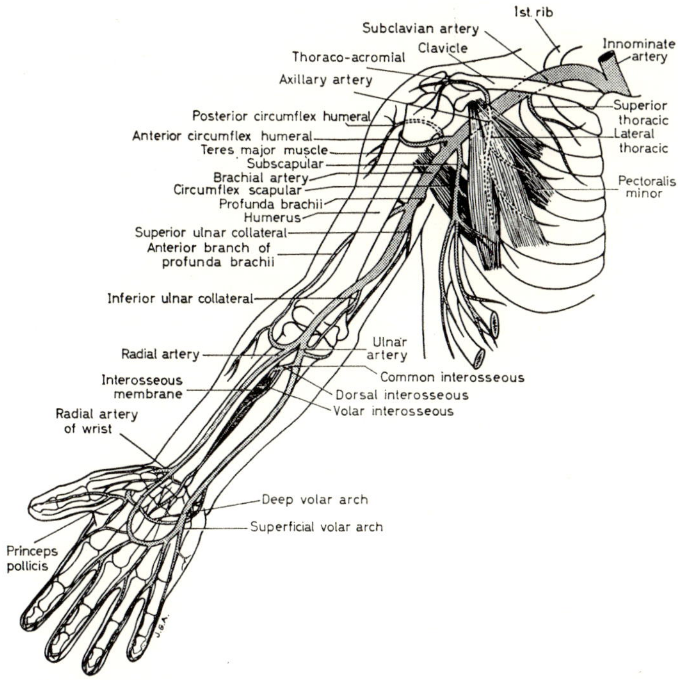

Figure 65. The arteries of the upper arm, forearm, and hand. As the subclavian artery passes through the armpit it becomes known as the axillary artery. In its course through the upper arm it is called brachial artery. It divides at the elbow into the ulnar and radial arteries.

throughout the body by smaller arteries. The muscular wall of the heart is called the *myocardium.*

CORONARY CIRCULATION. The myocardium or heart muscle must be supplied with blood, just as any other muscle of the body must. The blood which flows through the chambers of the heart is not absorbed by the muscle. The blood comes to the heart muscle through the *coronary arteries,* which are the first branches of the aorta.

THE LYMPHATIC SYSTEM. The lymphatic system consists of *lymphatic capillaries, lymphatic vessels,* and *lymph nodes.* The lymphatic capillaries are similar to blood capillaries and their function is to pick up tissue fluid and waste matter from the cells.

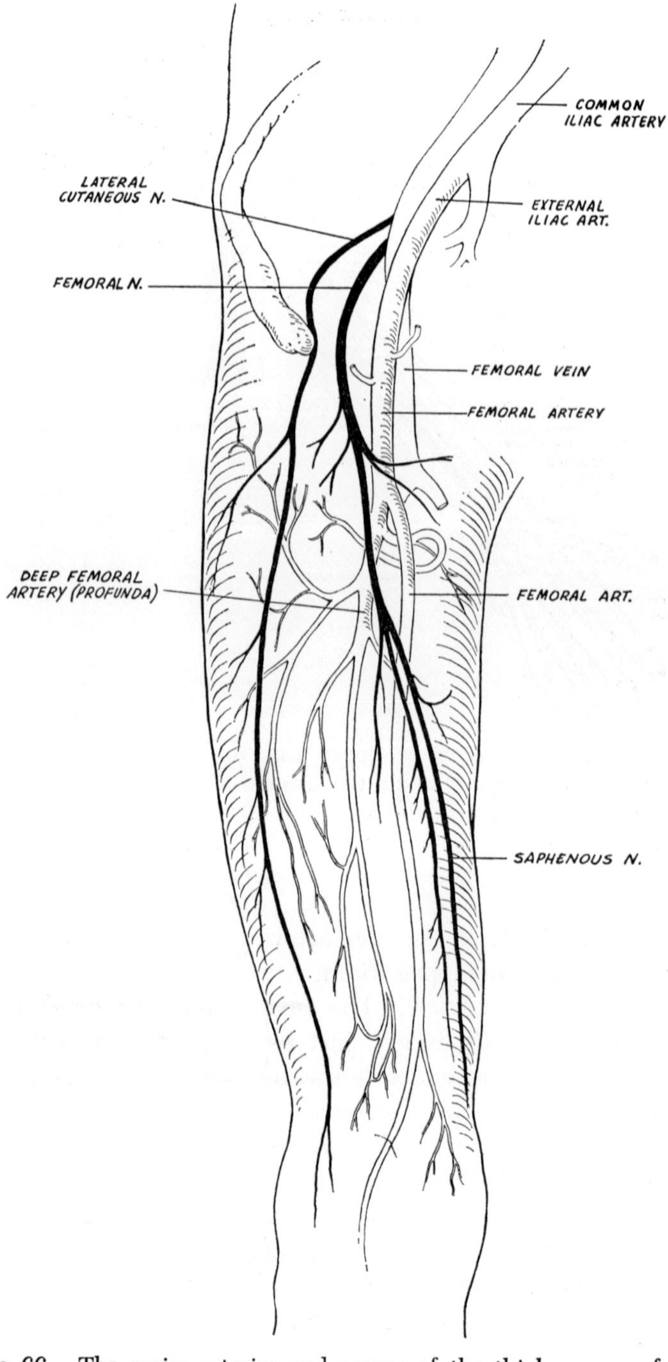

Figure 66. The major arteries and nerves of the thigh as seen from the front.

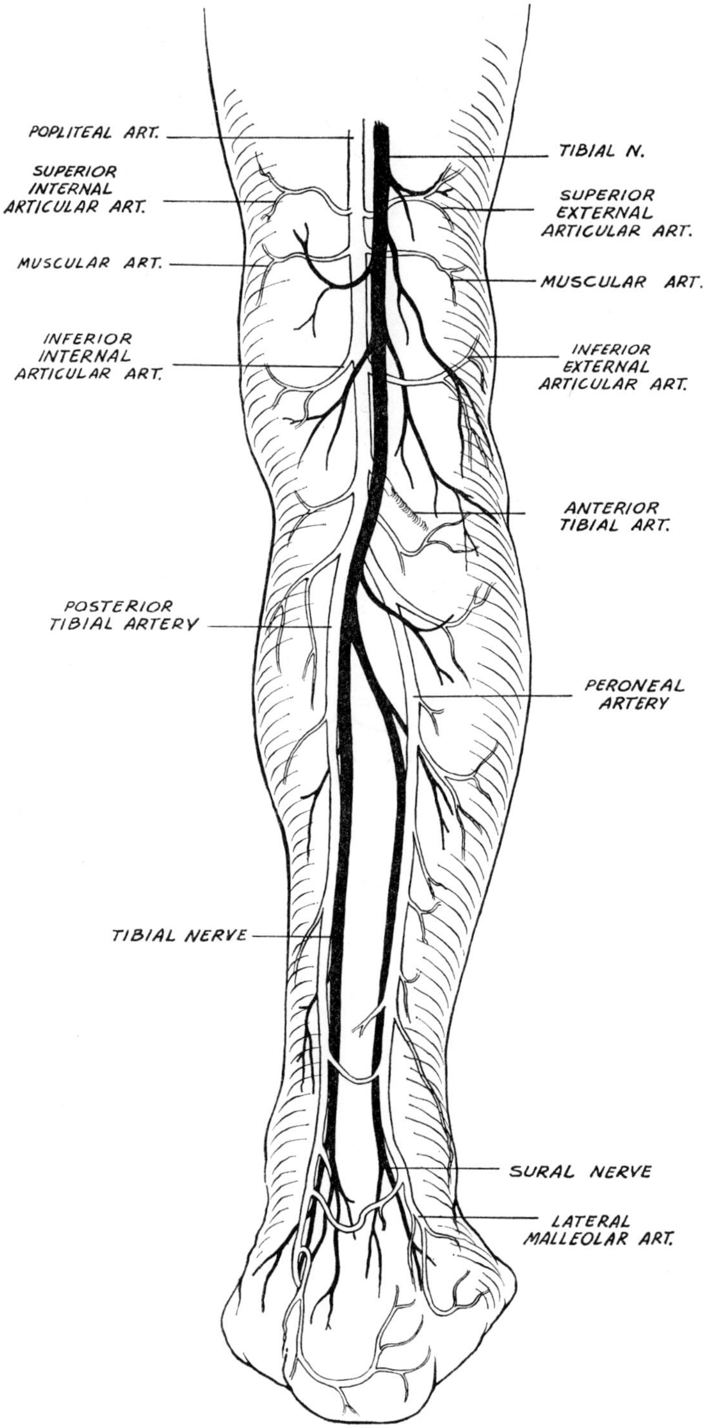

Figure 67. The major arteries and nerves of the leg as seen from the back.

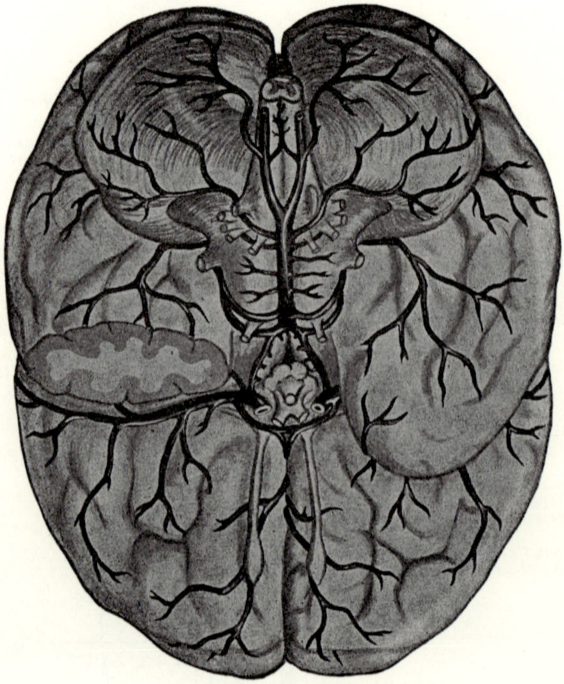

Figure 68. The circle of Willis, an arterial network seen on the underside of the brain.

The capillaries empty into progressively larger vessels, the lymphatic vessels. The system ends in two large vessels, the *thoracic duct* and the *right lymphatic duct*. These two vessels empty the lymph, as the tissue fluid is now known, into two large veins at the base of the neck. The lymph nodes are small masses of tissue situated at various points in the lymphatic system. The lymph nodes contain cells which destroy bacteria present in the lymph. They also act as filters. Another function of the nodes is the manufacture of monocytes and lymphocytes.

VOCABULARY REVIEW

Define the following terms on the basis of the preceding lesson. Consult a medical dictionary to determine the pronunciation.

aorta
arteries
atrium
auricle
basophils
bicuspid
capillaries
coagulation
coronary
endocardium
eosinophils
erythrocytes
granular
hemoglobin
leukocytes
leukocytosis
lymph nodes
lymphatic capillaries
lymphatic duct
lymphatic vessels
lymphocytes
mitral valve
monocytes
myocardium
neutrophils
nongranular
pericardium
plasma
platelets
thoracic duct
thrombocytes
tricuspid valve
veins
ventricle

VOCABULARY EXERCISE

With the aid of a medical dictionary, determine the etymologic composition of each of the following words:

basophil
bicuspid
coagulation
endocardium
eosinophil
erythrocyte
hemoglobin
leukocyte
leukocytosis
lymphocyte
monocyte
myocardium
neutrophil
pericardium
thrombocyte

What is the meaning of the following combining forms?

-phil
bi-
endo-
erythro-
hemo-
leuko-
-osis
mono-
myo-
-cardium

REVIEW QUESTIONS

1. What term describes the fluid portion of the blood?
2. What are the *erythrocytes* and *leukocytes?*
3. How do *arteries* differ from *veins?* What are *capillaries?*
4. What pigment gives the blood the characteristic red color?
5. What are the *eosinophils* and *basophils?*

6. Which of the formed elements of the blood help in coagulation?
7. What is the *pericardium?* What is the lining of the heart called?
8. What is an *atrium* and what is another name for it?
9. What is the lower chamber of the heart called?
10. What is the location of the *tricuspid* valve and *bicuspid* valve?
11. What is another name for the *mitral* valve? Where is it located?
12. What is the name of the largest artery of the body?
13. What is the *myocardium?* What does *myo-* refer to?
14. What is the name of the arteries supplying blood to the heart muscle?
15. What is meant by the *lymphatic system?*
16. What is the function of the *thoracic duct* and the right *lymphatic duct?*
17. What is the main function of the lymph nodes?

Chapter VIII

THE NERVOUS SYSTEM

FUNCTION OF THE NERVOUS SYSTEM. The main function of the system is the bringing of information and impressions from both within and without the body. Certain parts of the nervous system act as centers of coordination for the impressions coming from the internal and external environments. The system receives messages through *sensory nerves* and sends out messages through *motor nerves.*

STRUCTURE OF THE NERVOUS SYSTEM. The structural unit of the nervous system is the *neuron.* The neuron is to the nervous system what the brick is to the brick building. A neuron is a specialized cell. It consists of a *cell body,* the part containing the nucleus and the cytoplasm, and thread-like projections or *processes* known also as nerve fibers. These processes or fibers are of two kinds. The processes which carry impulses toward the cell body are the *dendrites.* Each neuron has several dendrites. The process which carries an impulse away from the cell body is called the *axon.* There is only one axon. On the basis of their function, neurons may be classified in three categories: *sensory* (conveying sensations), *motor* (conveying impulses causing muscular contraction), and *connecting* (which serve as intermediaries between other neurons). A nerve impulse may travel from the axon of one neuron to the dendrite of another. The junction of the two processes is called *synapse.*

DIVISIONS OF THE NERVOUS SYSTEM. The entire nervous system is subdivided into the *central nervous system, peripheral nervous system,* and the *autonomic nervous system.* The central nervous system is composed of the brain or *encephalon* and the *spinal cord* or *medulla spinalis.* The largest part of the encephalon or brain is the *cerebrum,* which occupies the upper part of the skull,

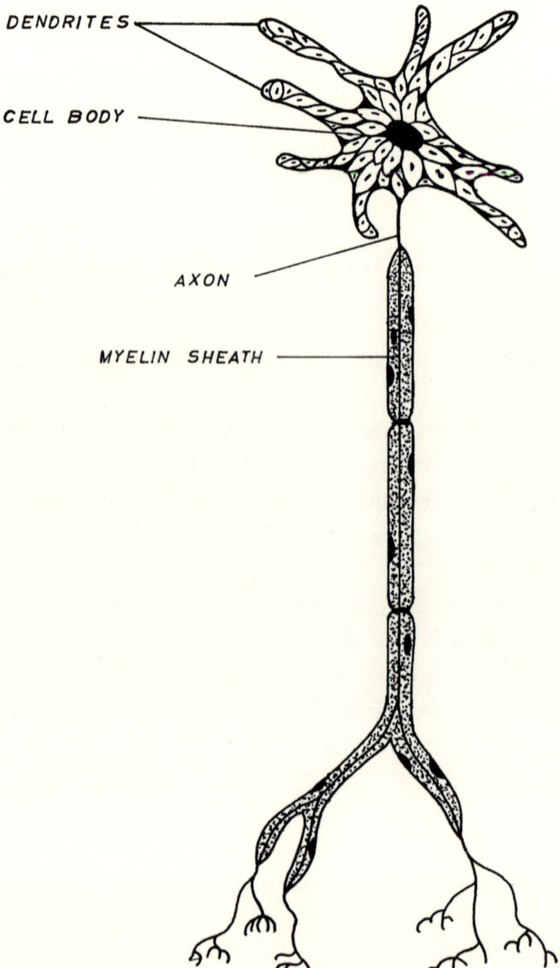

Figure 69. Diagram of a neuron or nerve cell, the structural unit of the nervous system. Note the cell body containing the nucleus without which the cell cannot live. The axon is surrounded by a sheath composed of a fatty substance called *myelin*.

i.e. the *cranium*. The cerebrum is divided into two halves, the right and left *hemispheres*. The superficial portion of the cerebrum is called *cortex*. It is also known as the *gray matter*. The cortex is divided into four lobes: *frontal, parietal, temporal,* and *occipital*. Beneath the two cerebral hemispheres are located two smaller brain structures: the *thalamus* and the *hypothalamus*.

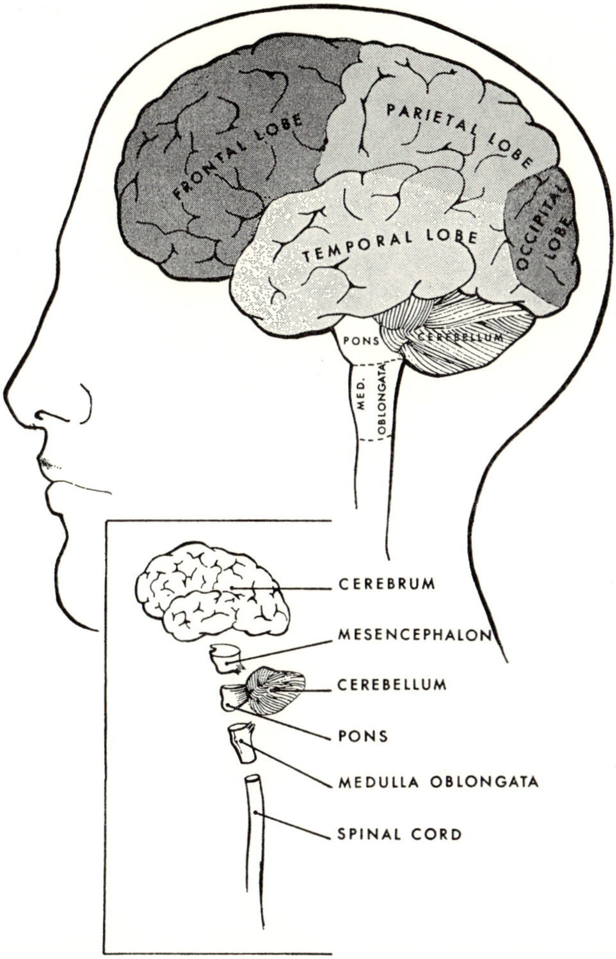

Figure 70. Side view of the brain and spinal cord showing the divisions of the brain and the lobes of the cerebrum.

The thalamus may be regarded as a relay station for nerve stimuli. The hypothalamus deals with heat regulation and water metabolism. The second largest part of the brain (next to the cerebrum) is called the *cerebellum.* It is located beneath the back part of the cerebrum. Its functions are concerned with muscle tone, coordination of muscular activity, and equilibrium. Beneath the cerebellum is the *brain stem,* a structure composed

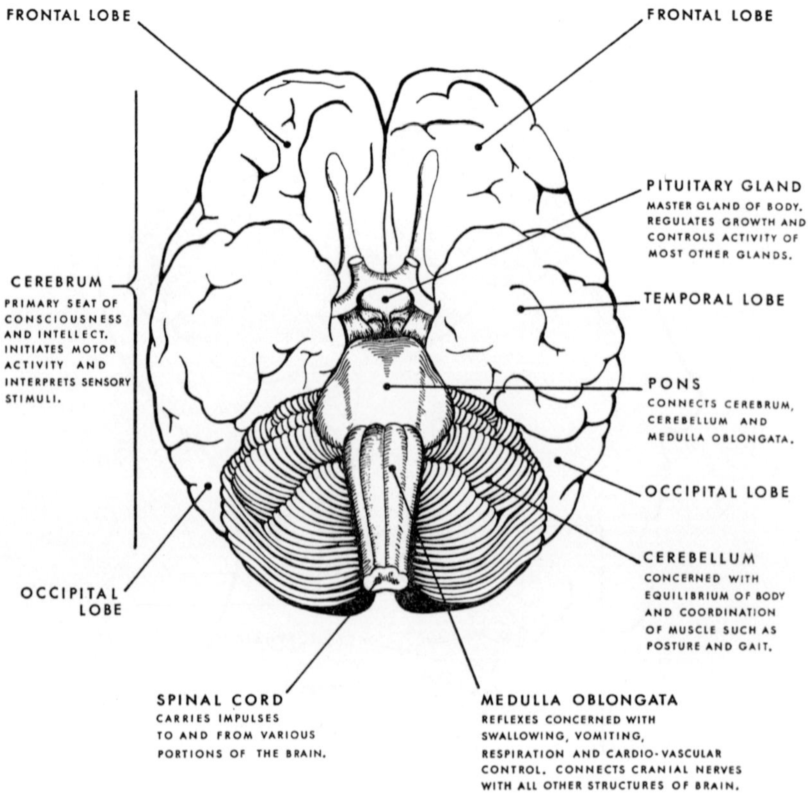

Figure 71. View of brain as seen from below. Note the functional importance of the various parts.

of the *midbrain*, the *pons*, and the *medulla oblongata*. The medulla controls many important functions of the body: the caliber of the blood vessels, the rate of the heart beat, the process of swallowing and breathing. The spinal cord is the cable of nerve cells and nerve fibers extending through a canal within the spinal column. It acts as a conduction pathway for impulses to and from the brain.

PERIPHERAL NERVOUS SYSTEM. This is composed of many nerves distributed through the muscles and skin. They are derived from two sources: from the 12 pairs of *cranial nerves*, which are joined directly with the brain (without the inter-

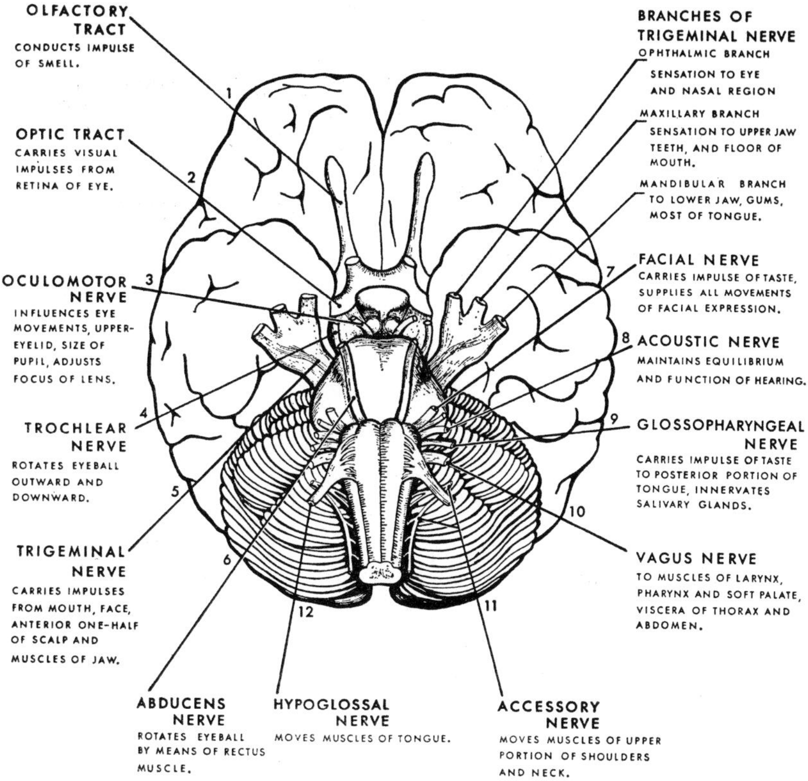

Figure 72. Functional "road map" of the cranial nerves (the nerves emerging directly from the brain), showing their distribution and the nature of their action.

mediacy of the spinal cord), and from the 31 pairs of *spinal nerves* (nerves which attach to the spinal cord). All of these carry such impulses as those concerned with pain, temperature, touch.

Autonomic Nervous System. This system is divided into two parts: the *sympathetic nervous system* and the *parasympathetic nervous system.* Both systems innervate smooth muscle (as the muscle of the stomach), the heart muscle, and the various glands. One system stimulates activity while the other system depresses or decreases activity. While the central nervous system functions consciously, i.e. is under the control of the will, the

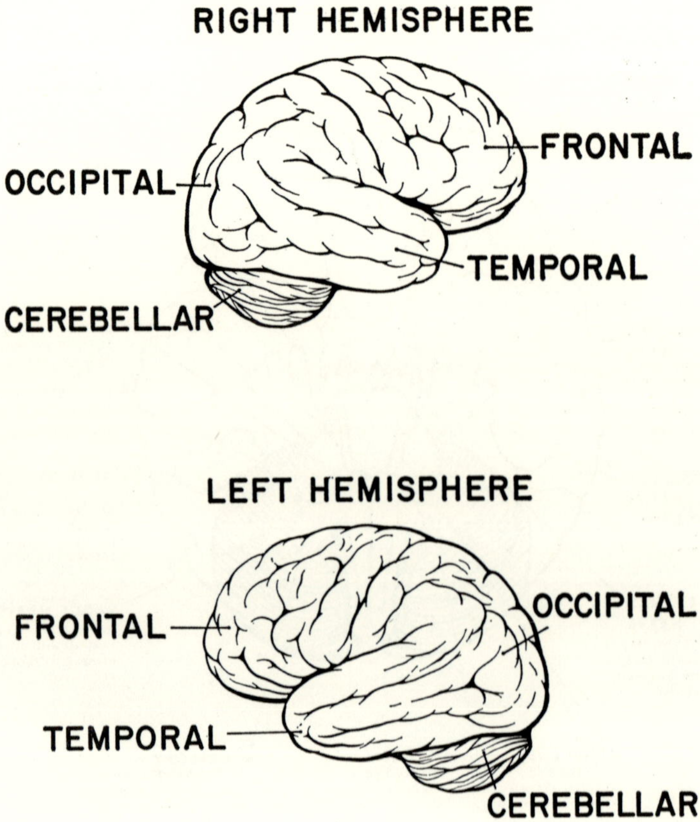

Figure 73. The hemispheres of the brain showing principal divisions.

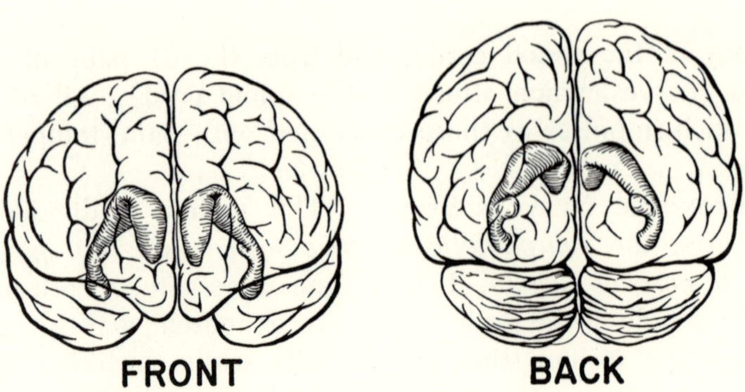

Figure 74. View of the brain showing the ventricles, where the cerebrospinal fluid is formed.

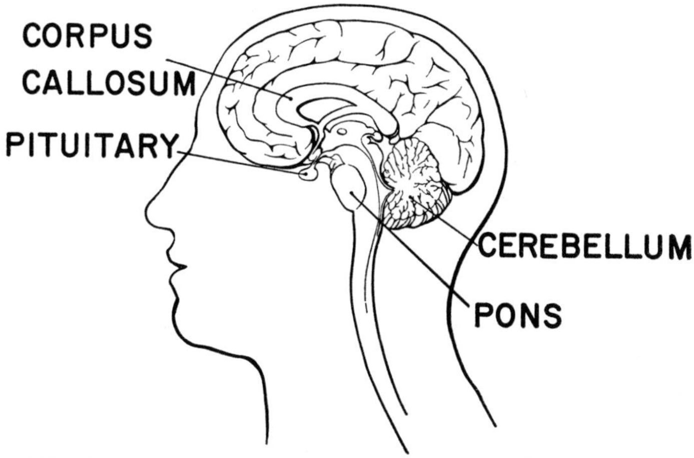

Figure 75. Diagram showing a sagittal section of the brain and its contents. Note position of pituitary gland.

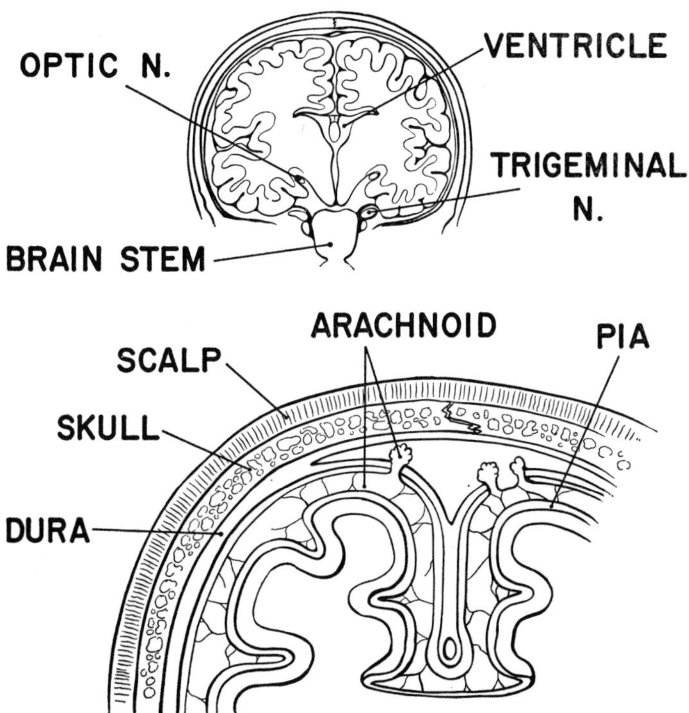

Figure 76. Frontal section of cranium and its contents. Note arachnoid (which secretes the cerebrospinal fluid) projecting into ventricles. Also note pia mater and dura mater.

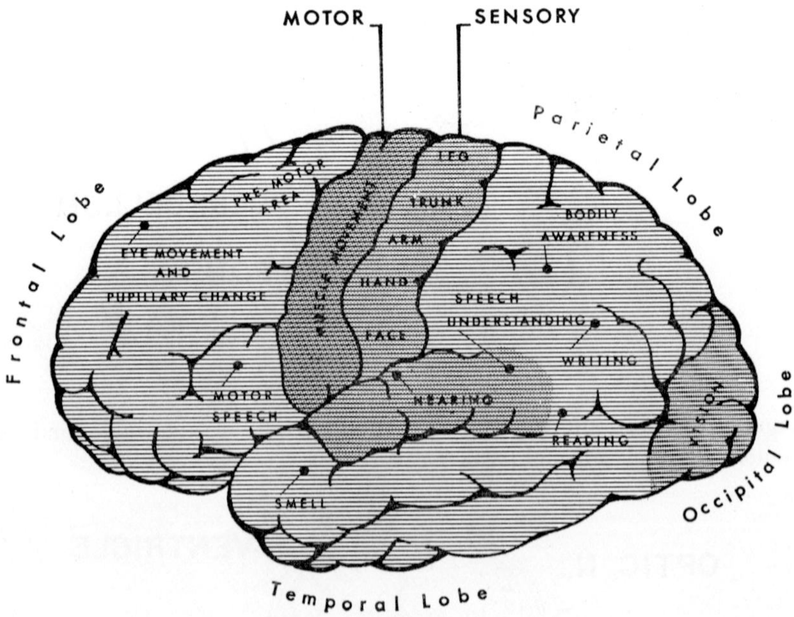

Figure 77. A "map" of the brain showing the various sensory and motor areas, i.e. the regions of the brain concerned with specific muscular action (as that involved in speech) and the perception of sensory stimuli.

autonomic nervous system is independent in its action. For example, the size of the pupil varies with the intensity of the lighting, but the adjustment takes place, without our willing it or our being conscious of it, through the agency of the autonomic nervous system.

The Reflex Arc. A sensory nerve impulse originating on the surface of the body begins at a *receptor,* a structure which is the initial receiver of the sensation (as heat or cold). The impulse travels through the dendrite and axon of a sensory nerve cell toward the spinal cord. It then passes upward through the cord and finally reaches the brain. The brain interprets the significance of the situation and, if an action is necessary, sends an impulse through another nerve, a motor nerve, in a direction opposite from the one received. If the sensation originated by the inadvertent touch of an excessively hot object, the reacting impulse

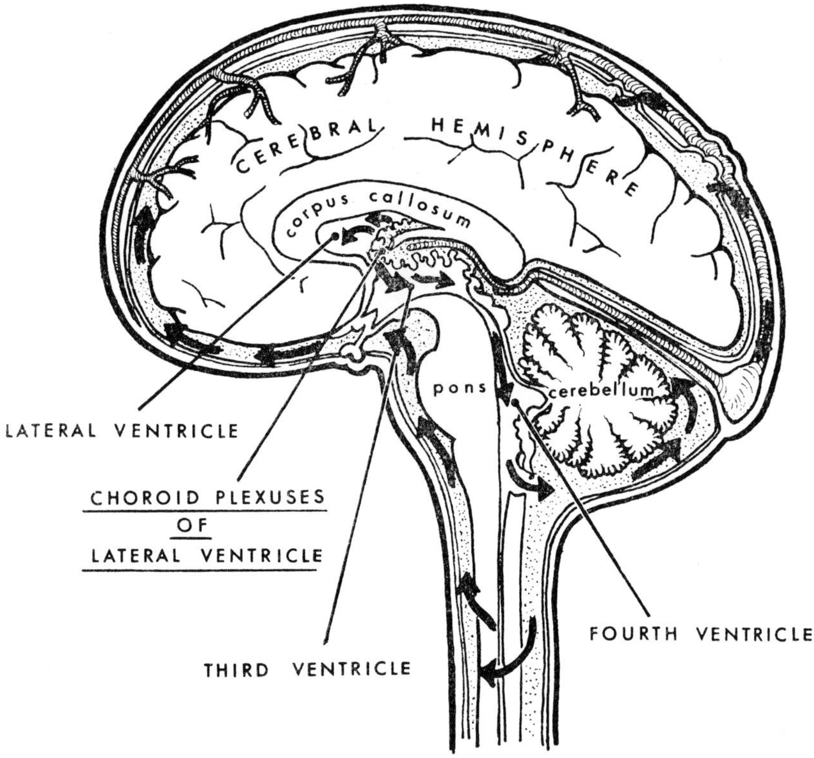

Figure 78. A cross-section of the cranium, showing the circulation of the cerebrospinal fluid in the subarachnoid space.

will cause certain muscles to contract and thereby remove the hand from the hot object. In certain cases, when the situation demands instantaneous action, the impulses which activate the muscles (for the withdrawal of the hand) begin to flow even before the sensory impulses reach the brain. This is accomplished by a kind of short circuit in the nerve pathway just described. As soon as the sensation of extreme heat reaches the spinal cord, a connecting neuron in the spinal cord causes an impulse to travel out of the spinal cord toward the muscles, via a motor nerve. Such an act is called a *reflex act;* the shortened pathway, which bypasses the brain, is known as a *reflex arc.*

THE CEREBROSPINAL FLUID. The brain and spinal cord of the

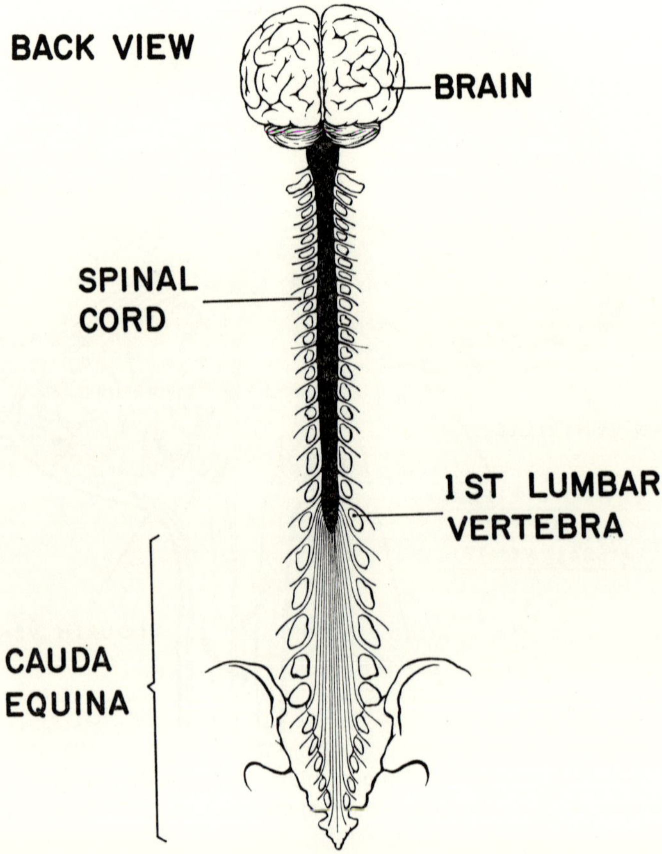

Figure 79. Back view of brain and spinal cord, showing the cauda equina, or horse's tail, a bundle of nerve fibers traveling in the lower part of the spinal cord.

central nervous system are covered by three protective membranes known as the *meninges*. These may be envisioned as a three-layered casing of a sausage. The innermost layer or membrane is the *pia mater*. It lies closely over the brain and the spinal cord. The next or middle layer is the *arachnoid*. There is a space filled with fluid between the pia mater and the arachnoid, called *subarachnoid space;* the fluid is known as the *cerebrospinal fluid*. The outermost of the three membranes is the *dura mater*. The singular of *meninges* is *meninx*.

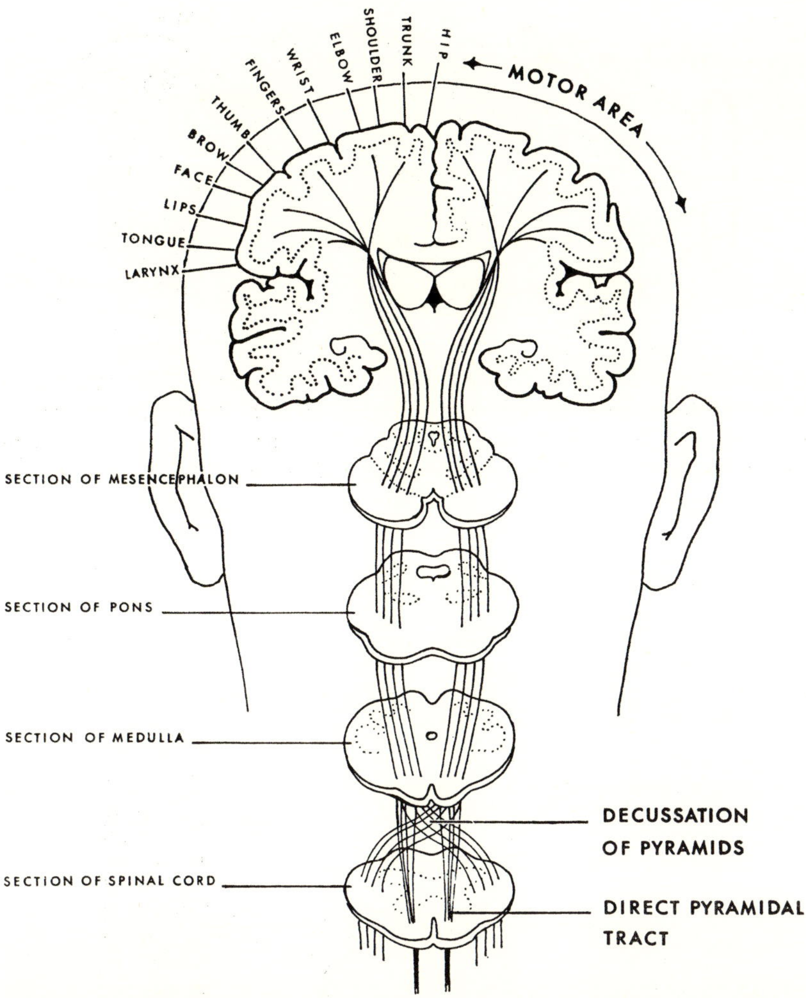

Figure 80. Schematic showing the decussation or cross-over of the pyramidal tracts, bundles of nerve fibers concerned with muscular movements.

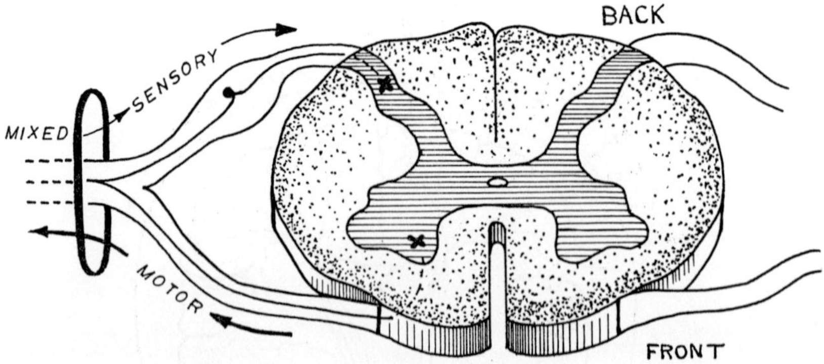

Figure 81. Diagram of a cross-section of the spinal cord. The dotted area is the white matter; the lines are the gray matter. Note that the motor nerve emerges from the front of the cord; the sensory nerve emerges from the back. The two roots merge into one mixed nerve.

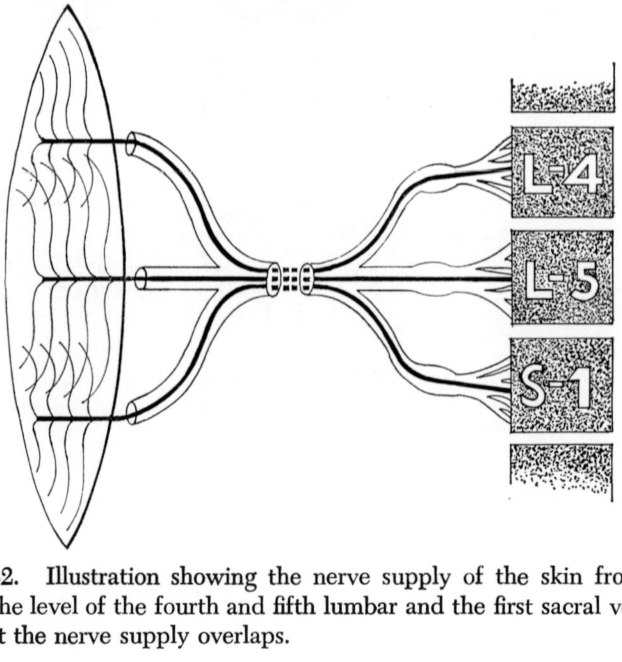

Figure 82. Illustration showing the nerve supply of the skin from nerve roots at the level of the fourth and fifth lumbar and the first sacral vertebrae. Note that the nerve supply overlaps.

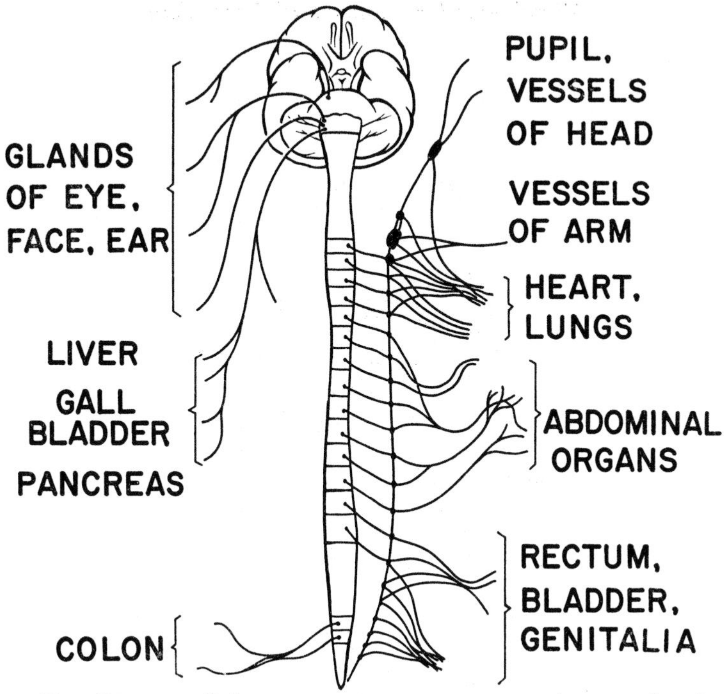

Figure 83. Diagram of the autonomic nervous system showing distribution to the principal organs.

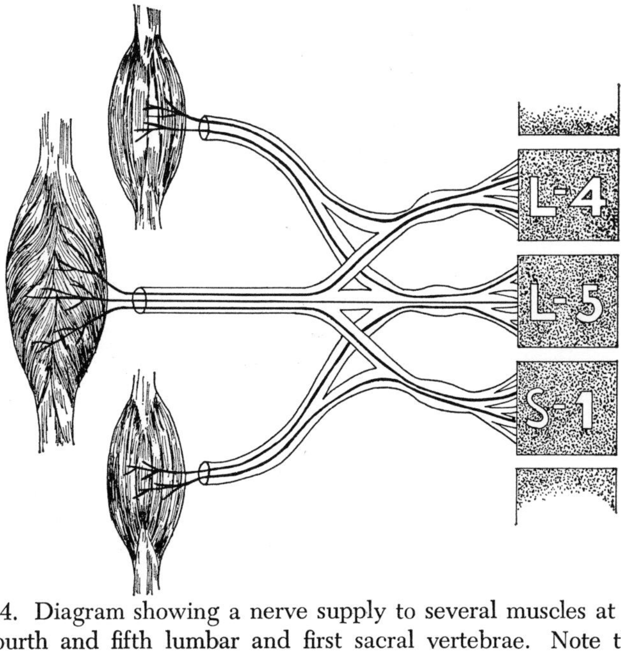

Figure 84. Diagram showing a nerve supply to several muscles at the level of the fourth and fifth lumbar and first sacral vertebrae. Note that each muscle receives nerve fibers from nerve roots at different levels.

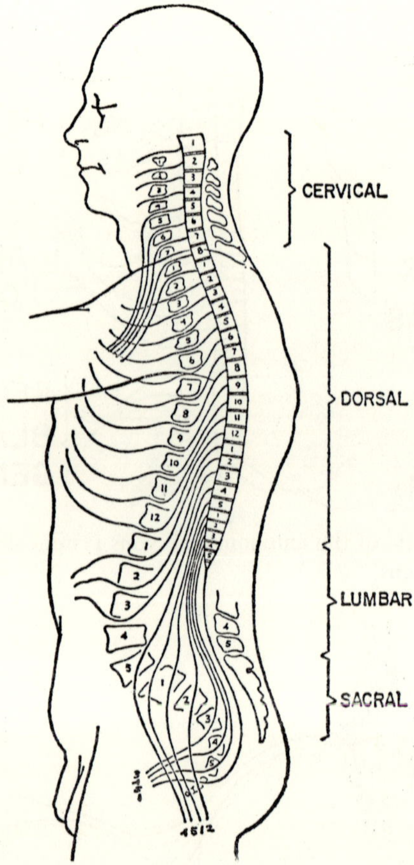

Figure 85. Diagram showing the bony levels of the spinal column and the corresponding levels in the spinal cord. Note that the nerves coming out between the lumbar and sacral vertebrae actually originate at a higher level of the spinal cord. Thus, the nerve at the fifth lumbar vertebra actually takes origin at the level of the twelfth thoracic vertebra.

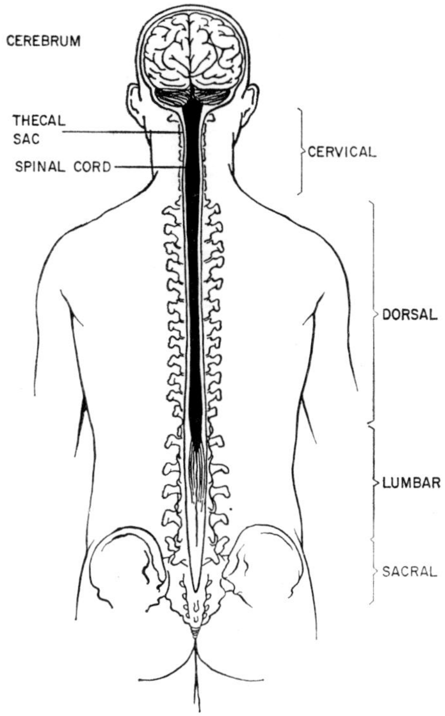

Figure 86. Posterior view of the central nervous system, i.e. the brain and spinal cord. Note that there is no cord below the level of the first lumbar vertebrae; however, the meninges extend lower and surround the cauda equina, the bundle of nerve fibers resembling a horse's tail.

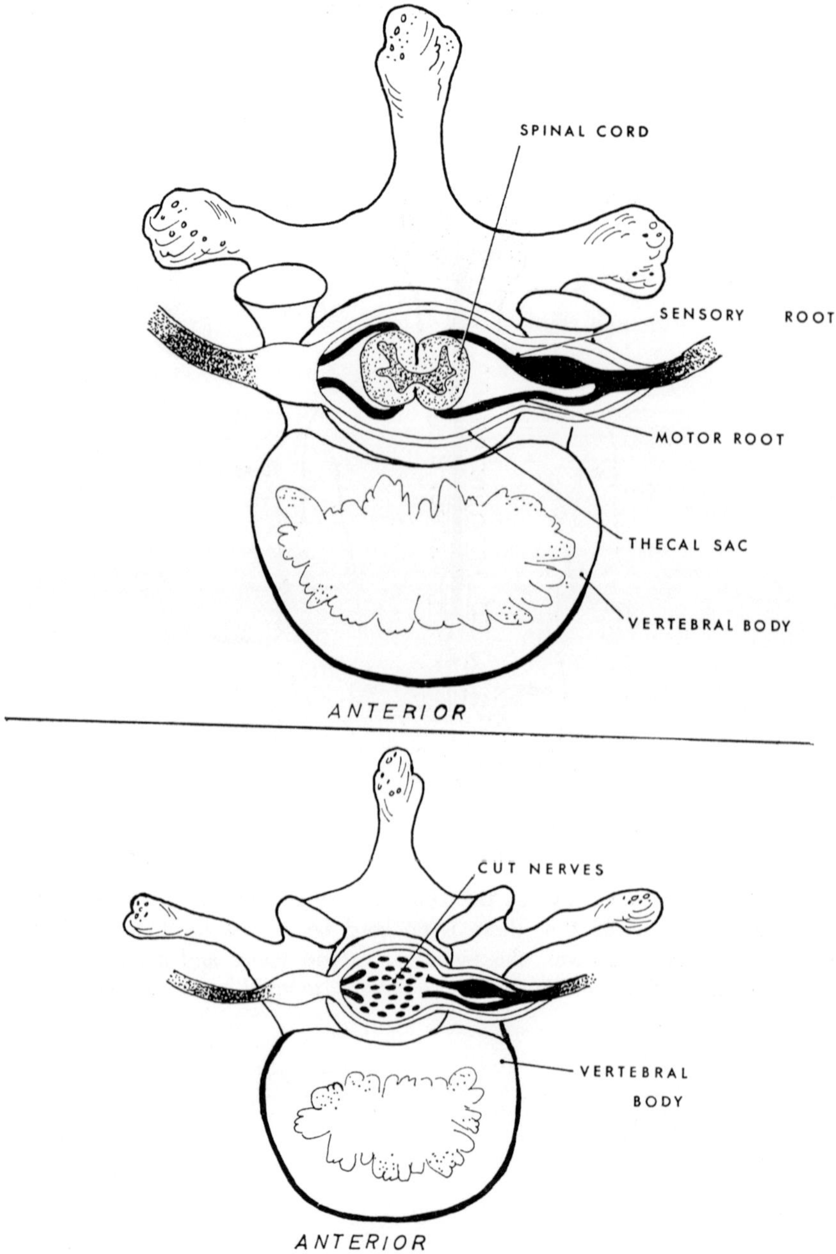

Figure 87. Cross-section of spinal column and cord about and below the level of the first lumbar vertebra. The lower diagram represents a level below the extent of the spinal cord. The dots represent the cut nerve fibers of the cauda equina, or "horse's tail," a bundle of nerves extending downward from the lowest segment of the spinal cord.

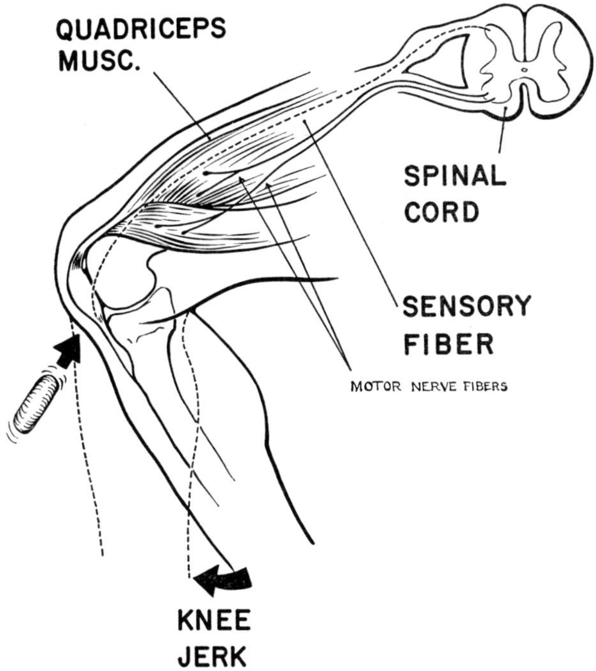

Figure 88. Schematic of the nerve pathway involved in the reflex arc of the knee jerk. When the kneecap is tapped, a nerve impulse is sent to the spinal cord through the sensory nerve. The impulse is relayed through the cord to the motor fibers which activate the quadriceps femoris muscle, which in turn causes the leg to kick up.

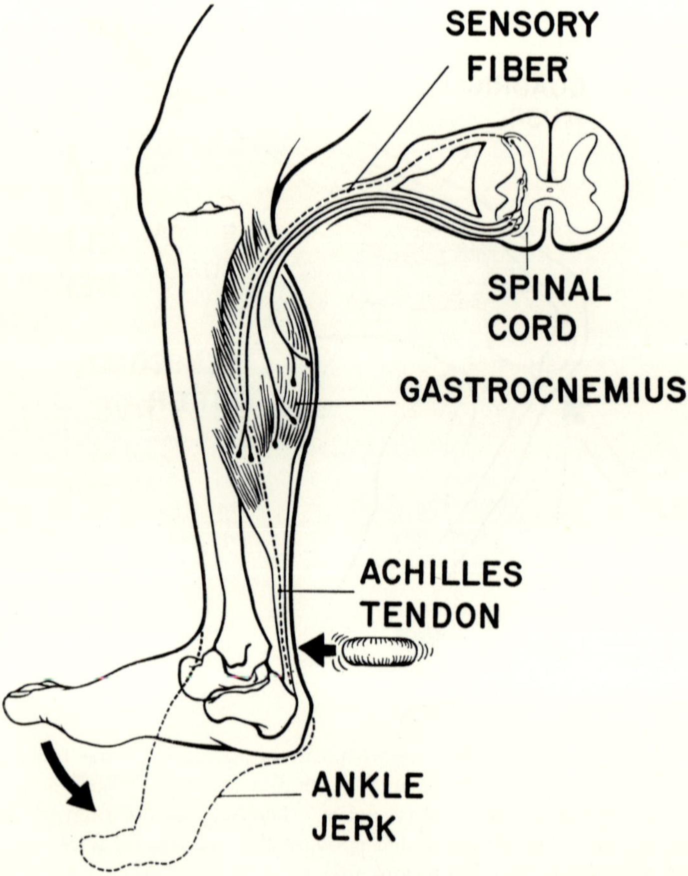

Figure 89. Nerve pathway in ankle jerk. When the Achilles tendon is tapped, a nerve impulse travels up the sensory nerve in the leg and thigh to the spinal cord, where it is relayed to the motor nerves of the calf muscles. This results in a sudden movement of the foot downward, the ankle jerk.

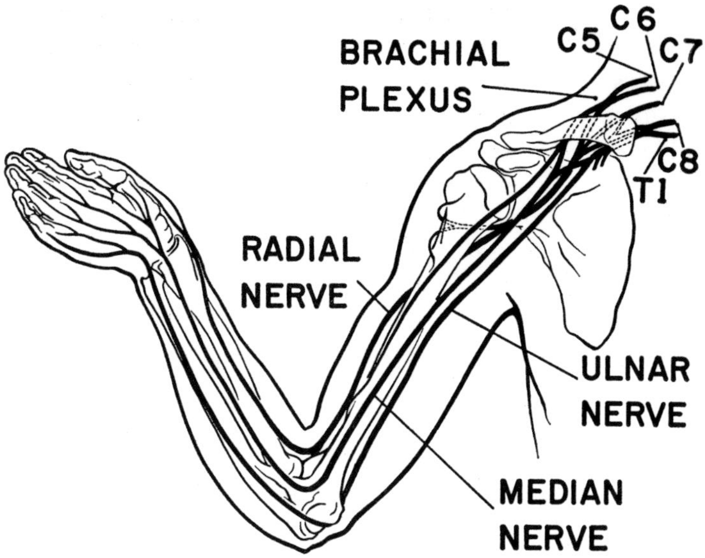

Figure 90. The principal nerves of the arm, known as the brachial plexus, derived from the fifth, sixth, seventh, and eighth cervical and first thoracic spinal nerves.

VOCABULARY REVIEW

Define the following terms on the basis of the preceding discussion. Consult a medical dictionary to determine the pronunciation.

arachnoid
autonomic nervous system
axon
brain stem
cell body
central nervous system
cerebellum
cerebrospinal fluid
cerebrum
connecting neurons
cortex
cranial nerves
cranium
dendrite
dura mater
encephalon
frontal lobe
gray matter
hemisphere
hypothalamus
medulla oblongata
medulla spinalis
meninges
meninx
midbrain
motor nerve
motor neuron
neuron
occipital lobe
parasympathetic nervous system
parietal lobe
peripheral nervous system

pia mater	reflex arc	sympathetic nervous system
pons	sensory nerves	synapse
process	sensory neuron	temporal lobe
receptor	spinal cord	thalamus
reflex act	spinal nerve	
	subarachnoid space	

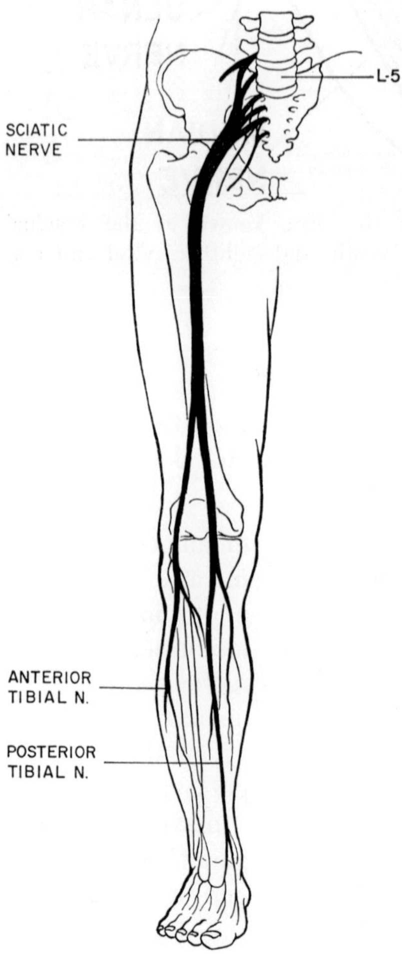

Figure 91. The sciatic nerve, the largest nerve of the body, originates in the fourth and fifth lumbar and the first, second and third sacral segments of the spinal cord. It innervates the muscles and skin of the lower extremity.

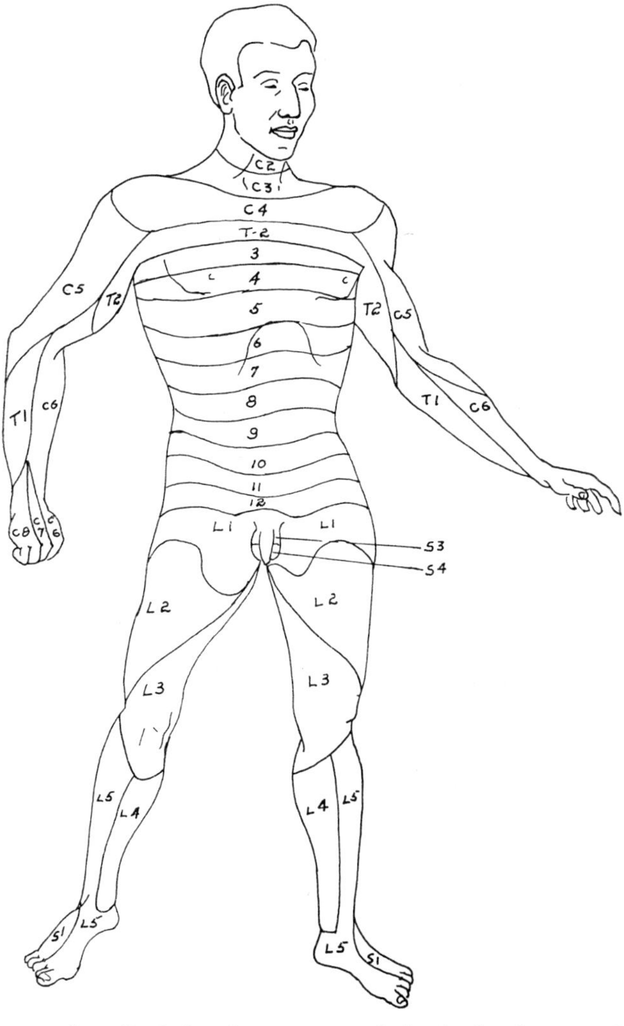

Figure 92. A "map" of the dermatomes of the body showing the nerve supply of each region. A dermatome is an area of skin supplied by the nerves of one sensory root of the spinal cord. Thus, the skin of the upper arm is supplied by the fifth cervical and second thoracic spinal nerves.

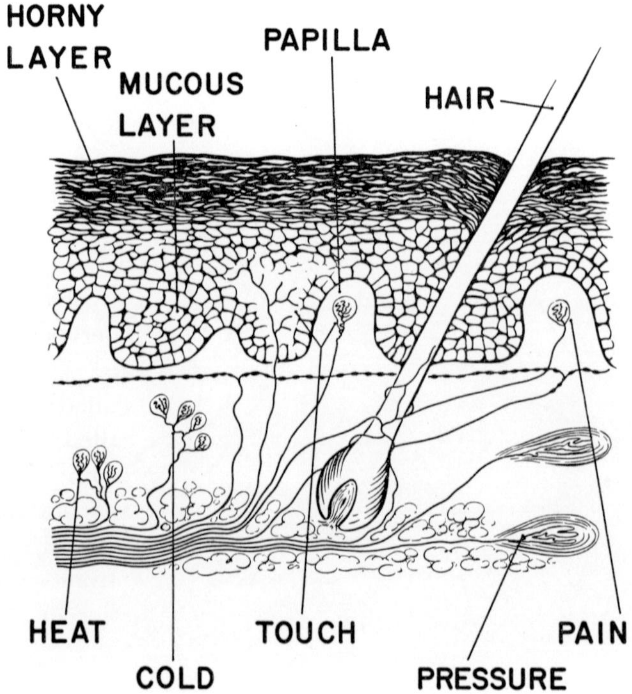

Figure 93. Microscopic cross-section of the skin showing distribution of the nerve endings for the reception of heat, cold, pain.

VOCABULARY EXERCISE

With the aid of a medical dictionary, determine the etymology of the following terms:

arachnoid	hemisphere
autonomic	hypothalamus
cerebrospinal	parasympathetic
dendrite	pia mater
dura mater	pons
encephalon	subarachnoid

REVIEW QUESTIONS

1. The nervous system receives "messages" through what nerves?
2. What are the nerves sending impulses to muscles?
3. What is the structural unit of the nervous system called?
4. What is a *neuron,* and what are its main structures or components called?
5. How does a *dendrite* differ from an *axon?*
6. What is a *synapse?* What structures does it involve?
7. What are the three main divisions of the nervous system?
8. What are the *encephalon* and *medulla spinalis?*
9. What is the largest subdivision of the brain called?
10. What is the superficial portion of the brain called?
11. What are the four lobes of the cortex of the brain?
12. What is the next to the largest portion of the brain called?
13. What are the component parts of the *brain stem?*
14. What is the name of the nerves emerging from the brain?
15. What are the subdivisions of the *autonomic nervous system?*
16. What is meant by reflex arc?
17. What are the names of the three meninges?
18. What is the name of the fluid in the subarachnoid space?

Chapter IX

THE DIGESTIVE SYSTEM

GENERAL CONSIDERATIONS. The energy required by the body to perform its various tasks is derived from foods. On the basis of chemical composition, the foods are divided into three classes: *carbohydrates* (comprising the sugars and starches), *proteins* (derived mainly from meats), and *fats* (derived from vegetable oils and the fats of animals). The function of the digestive system is to break food down into very small particles and to transform most of it into simple or simpler chemical substances. Thus, sugars and starches found in the food are changed chemically into simple forms of sugar that the body can utilize. Proteins are broken down into *amino acids.* Fats are changed into *fatty acids* and *glycerol* (commonly known as *glycerin*). In these simpler forms, the food passes from the digestive system to the circulatory system, by penetrating the walls of the digestive organs and the walls of the small blood vessels. The material is then distributed throughout the body by the circulating blood.

COMPONENTS OF THE DIGESTIVE SYSTEM. The entire digestive system may be envisioned as a continuous tube which begins with the mouth and ends with the anus. The food taken into the mouth is subjected to various physical and chemical changes, and as it moves along the tube (also known as the *alimentary canal* and *gastrointestinal tract*) the many useful components produced by the digestive process are withdrawn and utilized. The chemical changes associated with digestion are accomplished mainly by *enzymes,* complex chemical agents produced by the body. The chief component parts of the digestive system are the *mouth, pharynx, esophagus, stomach, small intestine, large intestine, biliary apparatus,* and *pancreas.*

The Mouth: The food enters the body through the mouth,

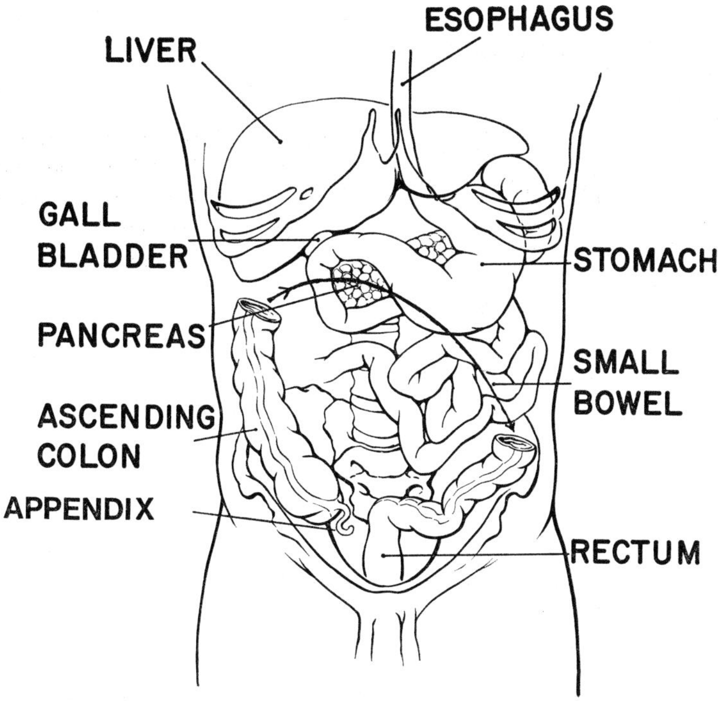

Figure 94. The principal digestive organs of the abdomen.

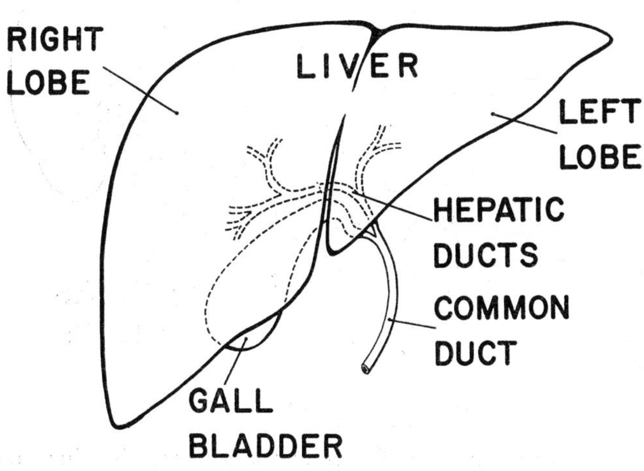

Figure 95. Diagram of liver and duct system.

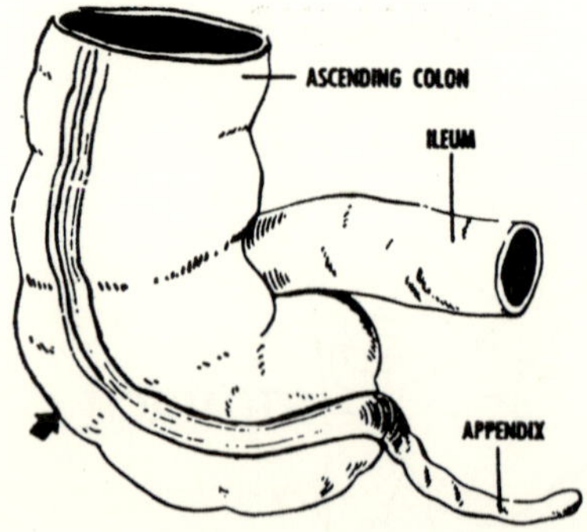

Figure 96. The junction of the small intestine with the colon. The portion of the colon below the entrance of the ileum is the cecum. Note position of vermiform appendix.

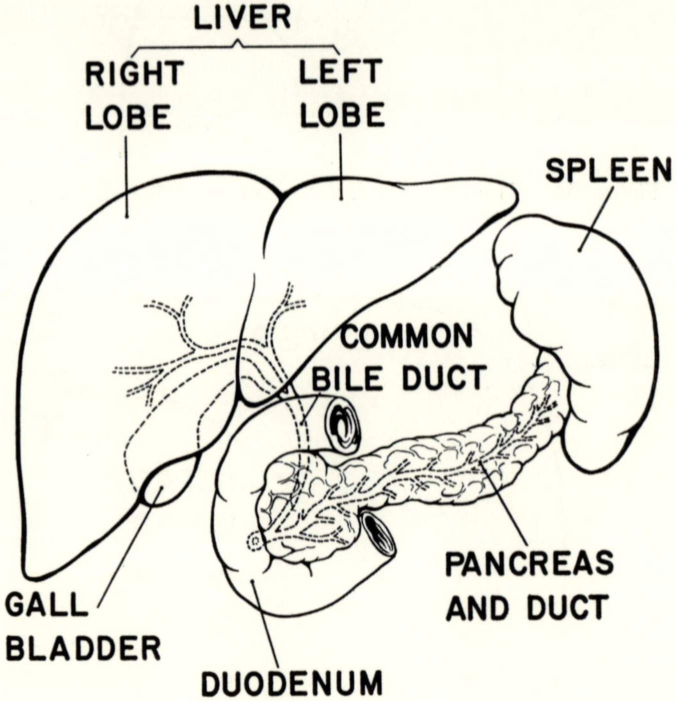

Figure 97. Diagram showing the pancreas between the duodenum and the spleen.

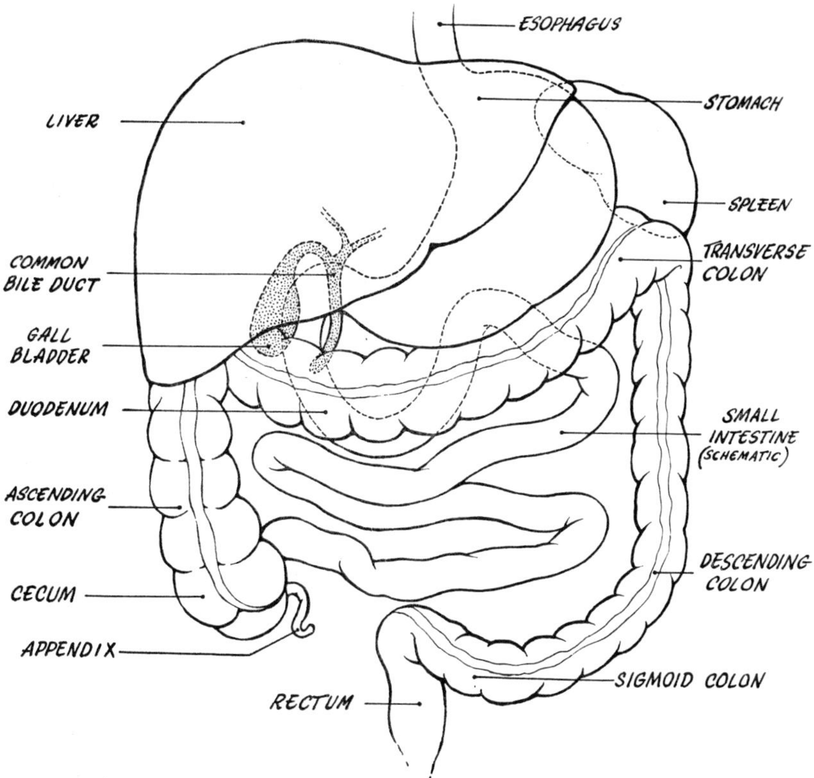

Figure 98. Schematic showing gastrointestinal tract, emphasizing the common bile duct, gallbladder, and large intestine or colon.

where it is cut up, ground, and mixed with saliva. The cutting and mixing process is accomplished by the teeth and tongue. The teeth, 32 of them in the adult, are set in *alveoli* or tooth sockets in the upper jaw—the *maxilla,* and the lower jaw—the *mandible.* The four front teeth, the *incisors,* are used to bite or cut. The tooth on each side of the incisors, the *canine,* is used for tearing. The back teeth, used for grinding, are the *molars.* Each tooth is composed of three anatomical parts: the *crown* (the part above the gum), the *root* (the part imbedded in the bone of the jaw), and the *neck* (the narrow part which joins the crown and the root at the gumline). The crown is covered

TRAUMA

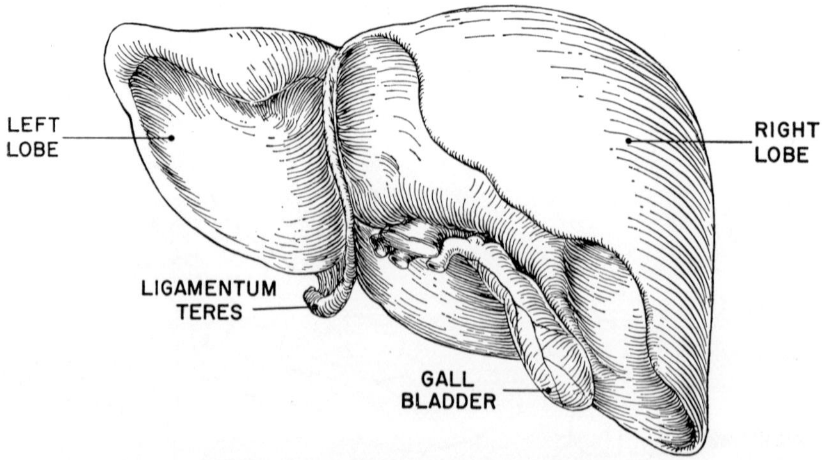

Figure 99. Posterior view of the liver.

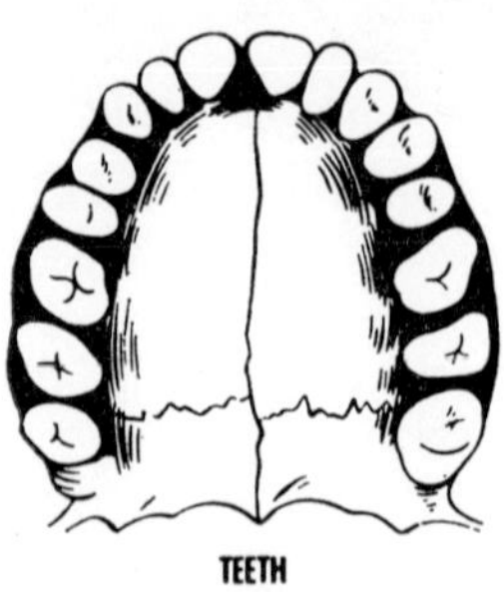

Figure 100. Upper teeth as seen from below. There are four incisors, two canines, four premolars, and six molars.

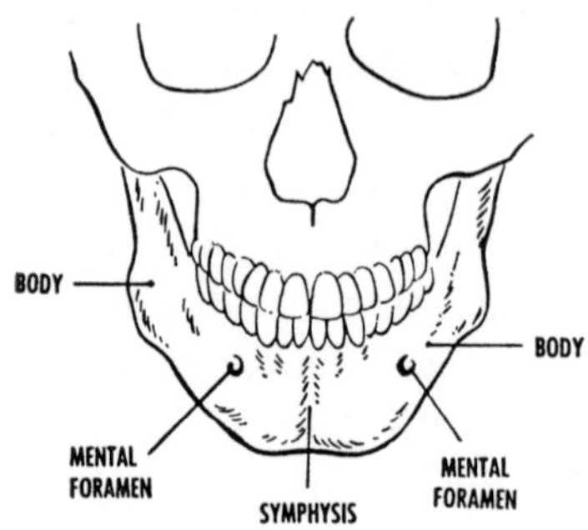

Figure 101. Front view of the mandible and maxilla (bone of upper jaw), showing upper and lower teeth.

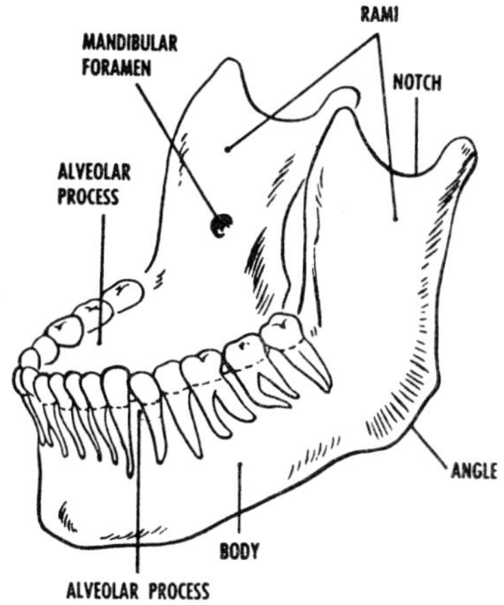

Figure 102. Anatomical parts of the mandible (bone of lower jaw).

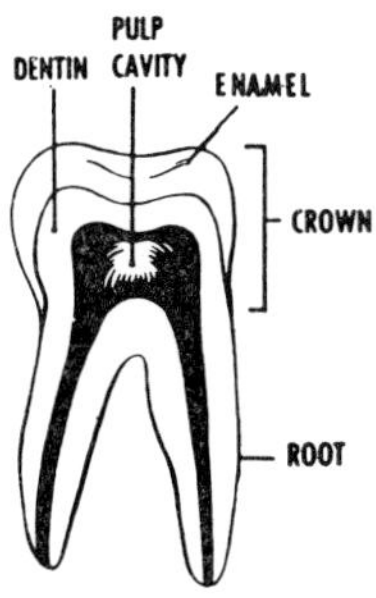

Figure 103. Cross-section of a molar tooth.

with *enamel,* the hardest substance of the body. The root and neck are covered with *cementum* or *cement.* The substance of the tooth under the crown and cementum is called *dentin.* In the center of the tooth is the vertical canal—the *pulp cavity,* which contains blood vessels and nerves (known collectively as the *pulp*).

The Tongue: The chewing or mastication of the food is helped by the movements of the *tongue,* a muscular structure covered with *mucous membrane* (a moist layer of tissue which also lines the mouth). The upper surface of the membrane shows numerous elevations called *papillae.* There are three types: *filiform papillae, fungiform papillae,* and *vallate papillae.* The *taste buds* (small organs containing nerve endings capable of distinguishing bitter, sweet, sour, and salty tastes) are distributed over the upper surface of the tongue, but they are most conspicuous on the sides of the vallate papillae (on the posterior part of the tongue).

The Salivary Glands: The saliva, which aids in softening the food, is produced by three pairs of *salivary glands*: the *parotid* (in front of and below the ear), the *submaxillary* (below the mandible), and the *sublingual* (under the tongue). The *saliva* is a thin watery fluid containing the enzyme *ptyalin* (also called *salivary amylase*), which acts on starch.

The Pharynx: A mass of food that has been chewed, mixed with saliva, and rolled by the tongue into a ball is called a *bolus*. The tongue starts the process of *deglutition* or swallowing by moving the bolus into the muscular tube behind the mouth, i.e. into the *pharynx*. The pharynx is often referred to as the throat. Contractions of the muscular walls of the pharynx propel the food into another muscular tube, the *esophagus*, which is a continuation of the pharynx.

The Esophagus: This may be visualized as a short length of garden hose (about 10 inches long) extending from the pharynx above to the stomach below. No digestion takes place in the pharynx and esophagus. These structures merely serve as passageways. The ring-like muscle of the esophagus at its junction with the stomach is the *cardiac sphincter*.

The Stomach: The stomach is a hollow, muscular, pear-shaped

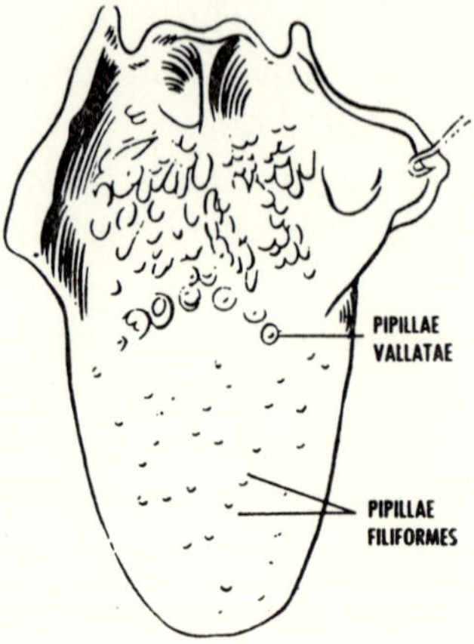

Figure 104. Dorsal view of the tongue showing the vallate and filiform papillae.

pouch situated in the upper part of the abdomen. The larger, rounded end, which is directed upward, is the *fundus*. The lower, tapering portion, which joins the small intestine, is the *pylorus* or *pyloric portion*. The central portion of the stomach, between the fundus and the pylorus, is the *body*. The muscular wall of the stomach consists of three layers of smooth muscle: an outer *longitudinal* layer, a middle *circular* layer, and an inner *oblique* layer. Its opening into the esophagus is the *cardiac orifice*. The opening into the small intestine is the *pyloric orifice*. The right border of the stomach (between these orifices) is the *lesser curvature*. It is relatively short and somewhat concave. The left border or *greater curvature* is convex and longer. The glands of the lining of the stomach secrete mucus and *gastric juice*, which consists of water, enzymes, and *hydrochloric acid*. The chief enzymes of the gastric juice are *pepsin* (which begins the breakdown of proteins) and *rennin* (which curdles the protein in milk). In the stomach, the food is churned into a semiliquid mass called *chyme*. In due time, the contractions of the muscular walls of the stomach move the chyme into the small intestine through the *pyloric outlet*, which is controlled by the *pyloric sphincter* (a muscle surrounding the pyloric outlet).

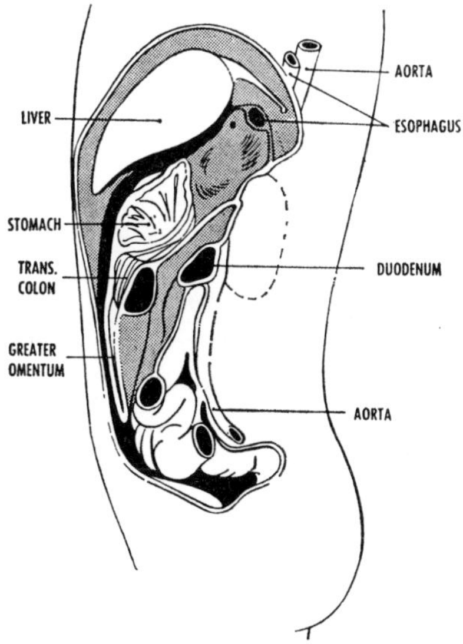

Figure 105. Diagram of sagittal section of the abdomen, showing relation of the internal organs to one another and to the greater omentum.

The Small Intestine: This is a tubular structure about 1½ inches in diameter and about 23 feet long. For descriptive purposes, it is divided into three parts: the *duodenum* (the first portion beginning at the outlet of the stomach), the *jejunum,* and the *ileum* (which joins the large intestine). As the food enters the duodenum, more digestive juices are added. The *bile,* which is produced in the liver, acts on fats. The pancreas adds three enzymes: *protease* (acting on proteins), *amylase* (acting on carbohydrates), and *lipase* (for the digestion of fats). As the food is being digested, rhythmic contractions of the muscular coats of the intestinal wall move the material forward, through the jejunum and ileum. Finger-like projections from the lining of the intestine, called *villi,* absorb the prepared food as it moves. Each *villus* (singular of *villi*) has an abundant supply of blood vessels and a lymph channel called *lacteal.*

The Large Intestine: This tubular structure is about 2½ inches in diameter and about 5 feet long. It is divided into the *cecum* (which has a closed or blind beginning), the *colon,* and the *rectum.* The cecum, which begins on the right side of the lower abdomen, has a wormlike projection, the *vermiform appendix* (the inflammation of which is called *appendicitis*). The small intestine empties into the large intestine at the junction of the cecum with the colon. The colon is divided into four parts: the *ascending colon,* the *transverse colon,* the *descending colon,* and the *sigmoid colon* (which is on the left side of the abdomen and is continuous with the next part, the rectum). The lower end of the rectum terminates as the *anal canal,* whose opening to the outside is the *anus.* By the time the digested food reaches the rectum, it consists of semisolid waste known as *feces.* The act of expelling the feces is called *defecation.* It should be noted that the food is propelled through the entire length of the digestive tract by a type of contraction which is preceded by a relaxation of the muscular walls of the tract. The movement is known as *peristalsis.* The term "feces" is plural in form.

Accessory Digestive Organs: The digestive process is augmented by the salivary glands (already mentioned), the *liver,* and the *pancreas.* The liver is the largest organ of the body. It is composed of a *right lobe* and a *left lobe.* The cells of the liver

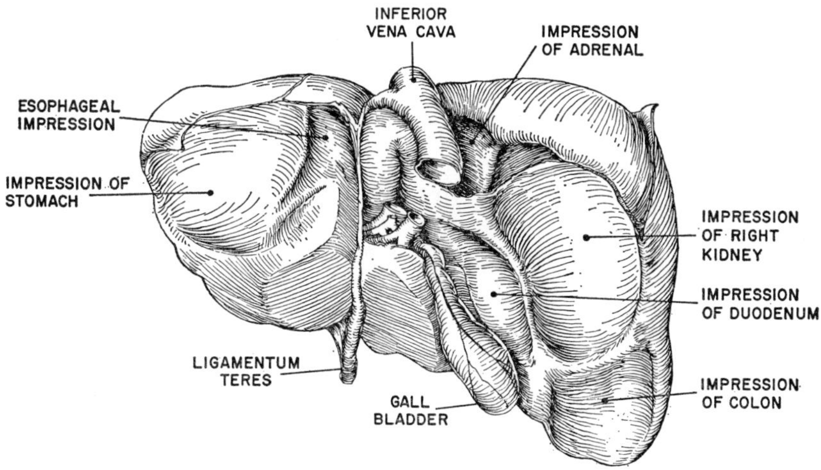

Figure 106. Liver as seen from below and behind.

are arranged in units called *lobules*. Blood is brought to the liver from two sources: from the digestive tract by the *portal vein* and from the aorta by the *hepatic artery*. One of the functions of the liver is the formation of bile. Small *bile ducts* emerge from the liver and join to form the *hepatic duct*, which carries the bile to the duodenum and, by way of the *cystic duct*, to the *gall-bladder*. The structures concerned with the formation, storage, and conduction of the bile are known collectively as the *biliary apparatus*. Under certain conditions the bile is absorbed by the blood, causing *jaundice* or *icterus*. It is marked by a yellow pigmentation of the skin. Sometimes the bile solidifies into *gallstones* or *biliary calculi*. A biliary calculus may cause severe pain (*biliary colic*).

The Pancreas: This organ lies in the abdomen, behind the stomach. It produces two kinds of secretion: the *pancreatic juice* for the digestion of food (discussed above) and *insulin* (which the body needs for the *metabolism* or utilization of sugars). The pancreatic juice is carried to the duodenum by a duct, the *pancreatic duct*. The insulin is produced by masses of cells known as *islets of Langerhans;* it is distributed without the aid of ducts by the circulating blood.

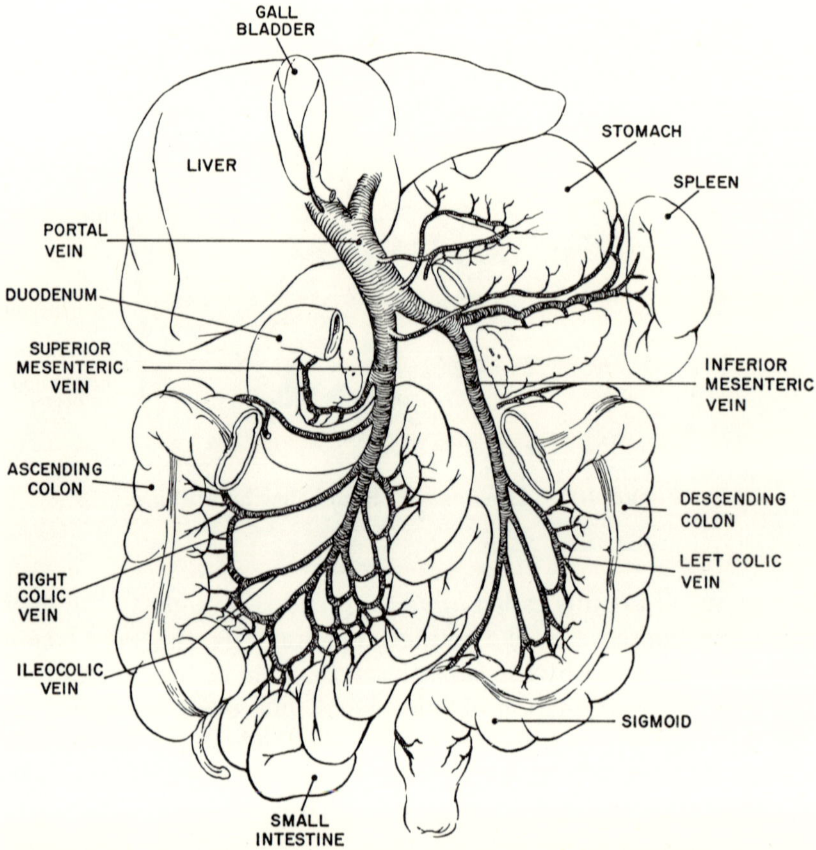

Figure 107. The portal vein and its tributaries carrying blood from the digestive organs to the liver.

The Peritoneum: The inner surface of the abdomen is covered by a *serous membrane* called *peritoneum*. It has the same relation to the walls of the abdomen as wallpaper has to the walls of a room. The peritoneum also covers the surfaces of the organs within the abdomen. A fold of peritoneum supporting the intestine is called *mesentery*. A fold of peritoneum extending between the stomach and the liver is the *lesser omentum*. The *greater omentum* is a large fold of peritoneum which spreads over the intestines like an apron.

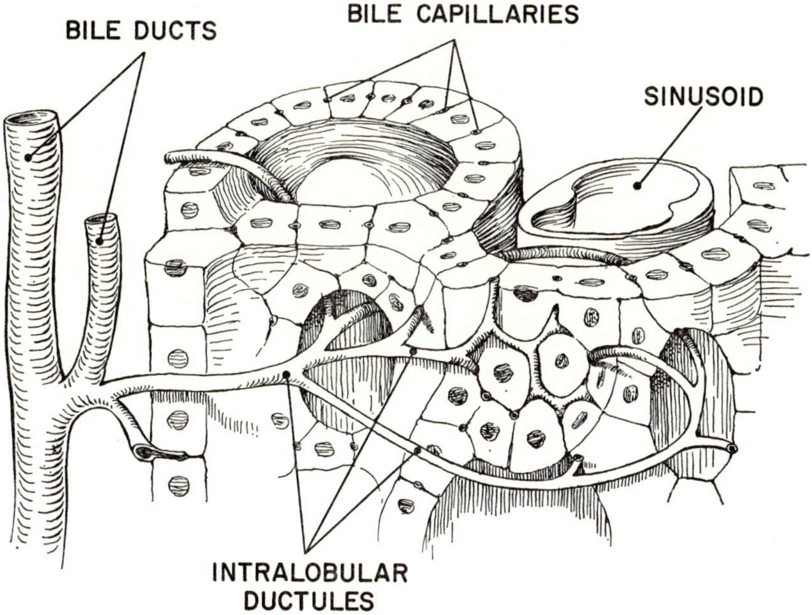

Figure 108. Diagram of the microscopic structure of the liver, showing bile ducts, bile capillaries.

VOCABULARY REVIEW

Define the following terms on the basis of the preceding discussion. Consult a medical dictionary for the pronunciation.

alimentary canal
alveoli
amino acid
amylase
anal canal
anus
appendicitis
ascending colon
bile
bile duct
biliary apparatus
biliary calculi
biliary colic
body
bolus
canine
carbohydrate
cardiac orifice
cardiac sphincter
cecum
cement
cementum
chyme
circular layer
colon
cystic duct
defecation
deglutition
dentin
descending colon
duodenum
enamel
enzyme
esophagus
fats
fatty acids

feces
filiform papillae
fundus
fungiform papillae
gallbladder
gallstones
gastric juice
gastrointestinal tract
glycerin
glycerol
greater curvature
greater omentum
hepatic artery
hepatic duct
hydrochloric acid
icterus
ileum
incisor
insulin
islets of Langerhans
jaundice
jejunum
lacteal
large intestine
left lobe
lesser curvature
lesser omentum
lipase
liver
lobule
longitudinal layer
mandible
maxilla
mesentery
metabolism
molar
mucous membrane
neck
oblique layer
pancreas
pancreatic duct
pancreatic juice
papillae
parotid gland
pepsin
peristalsis
peritoneum
pharynx
portal vein
protease
protein
ptyalin
pulp
pulp cavity
pyloric orifice
pyloric outlet
pyloric portion
pyloric sphincter
pylorus
rectum
rennin
right lobe
root
saliva
salivary amylase
salivary gland
serous membrane
sigmoid colon
small intestine
sublingual gland
submaxillary gland
taste buds
tongue
transverse colon
vallate papillae
vermiform appendix
villi
villus

VOCABULARY EXERCISE

Using a medical dictionary as a reference, answer the following questions:

1. What does *alimentary* refer to?
2. What is the singular of *alveoli*?
3. What does the suffix *-ase* mean?
4. What does *-itis* indicate?
5. What is the singular of *calculi*?

6. What are the components of *carbohydrate?*
7. What is *defecation* derived from?
8. What is the story behind *duodenum?*
9. What does *filiform* mean?
10. What is the meaning of *fungiform?*
11. What does *gastro-* mean?
12. What does *hydrochloric* mean?
13. Why is *jejunum* so named?
14. What is the etymology of *peritoneum?*
15. What does *pyloric* mean?
16. Why is the *rectum* so called?
17. What does *sigmoid* mean?
18. What does *vermiform* mean?

REVIEW QUESTIONS

1. What are the three classes of food?
2. Proteins are broken down into what acids?
3. Into what substances are fats broken down?
4. What is another name for the *alimentary canal?*
5. What do the *maxilla* and *mandible* have in common?
6. What are the *incisors, canines,* and *molars?*
7. What are the principal anatomical parts of a tooth?
8. Where do you find *dentin, cementum, enamel?*
9. With regard to a tooth, what is meant by *pulp?*
10. What is the medical word for *chewing?*
11. What kinds of *papillae* are found on the tongue?
12. What enzyme does the saliva contain?
13. What salivary glands are found in the mouth?
14. A mass of chewed food ready for swallowing is called what?
15. What is the medical term for *swallowing?*
16. What is the medical name for the *gullet?*
17. What lies between the back of the mouth and the esophagus?
18. Where is the *cardiac sphincter?*
19. What are the anatomical divisions of the *stomach?*
20. What medical combining form refers to the *stomach?*
21. Where is the *pyloric sphincter?*
22. What are the three divisions of the *small intestine?*

23. Which of the enzymes aids in the digestion of fats?
24. What are the finger-like projections from the intestine called?
25. What is the medical term for the *large intestine?*
26. Into what parts is the *colon* divided?
27. Can you name the movement which propels the food?

Chapter X

THE RESPIRATORY SYSTEM

GENERAL CONSIDERATIONS. The cells of the body must have a sufficient supply of *oxygen* in order to live. The source of the oxygen is the air that we breathe. The air is taken into the body through the lungs by the process of *respiration* or breathing. Respiration also serves to eliminate *carbon dioxide,* a waste product of body cells. A cycle of respiration consists of two phases: an *inspiration* or inhaling (during which the air is drawn into the lungs) and an *expiration* or exhaling (during which air laden with carbon dioxide is expelled from the lungs).

THE RESPIRATORY APPARATUS. The anatomical structures in-

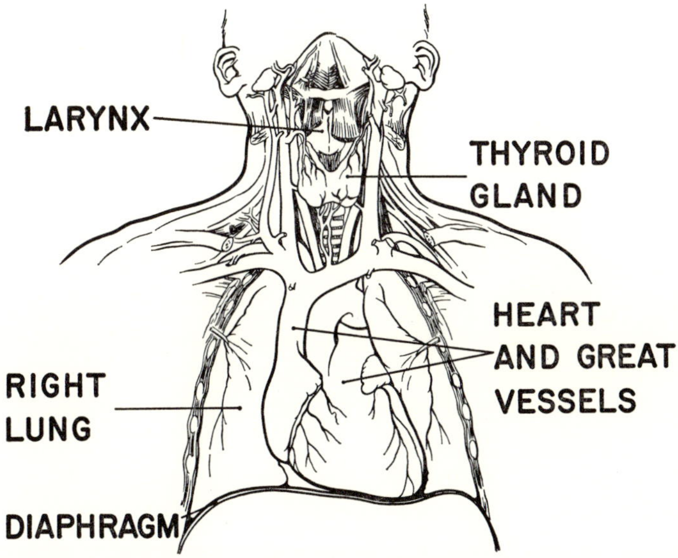

Figure 109. A dissection of the front of the chest and neck showing relation of the heart, lungs, and the great blood vessels.

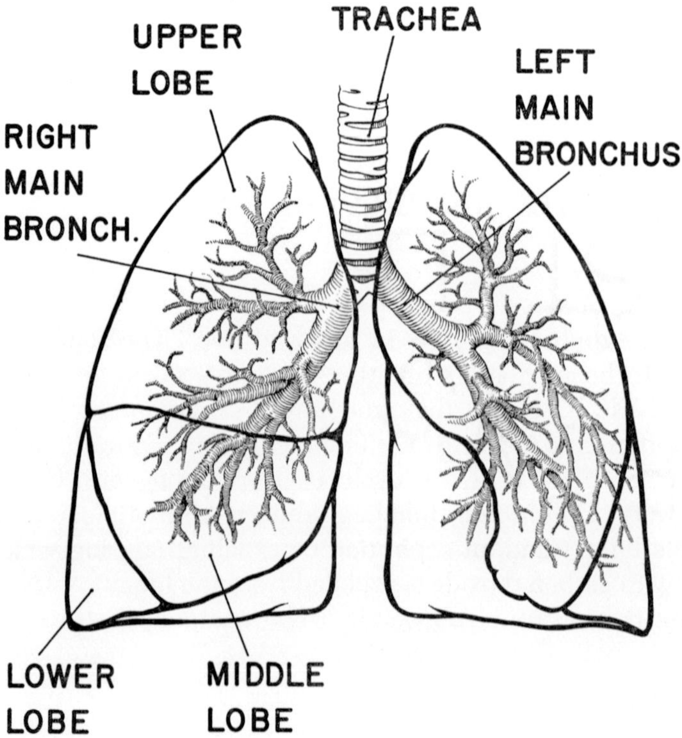

Figure 110. Schematic anterior view of the lungs, trachea, and the bronchi.

volved in respiration are the nose, pharynx, larynx, trachea, bronchi, bronchioles, alveoli, respiratory muscles, blood vessels, and nerves. Normally, air begins its passage into the body through the nose. The interior of the nose is lined with mucous membrane, which aids in moistening, warming, and cleansing the air before it reaches the lungs. The *vibrissae* (the hairs at the nostrils) and the *cilia* (hair-like projections on the mucous membrane) also help in removing dust and other particles from the air.

The Pharynx: The inhaled air moves through the back openings of the nose (the *posterior nares* or the *choanae*) into the upper part of the pharynx (the *nasopharynx*) and down to the *larynx* or voice organ. The part of the pharynx below the level

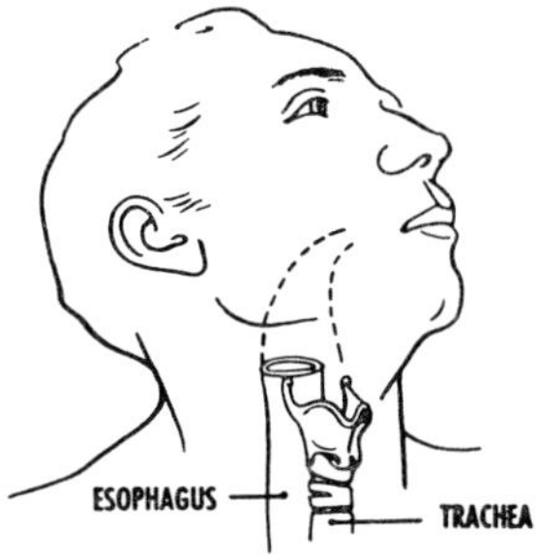

Figure 111. Diagram showing relation of trachea to esophagus.

of the roof of the mouth is the *oropharynx.* The *adenoids,* a mass of lymphoid tissue, are located in the nasopharynx. The *tonsils* (two masses of lymphoid tissue) are located in the oropharynx, one on each side.

The Larynx: The voice organ with its central opening (which leads into the *trachea* or windpipe) is situated in the front wall of the lower part of the pharynx (where the pharynx ends and the esophagus begins). To prevent food from entering the opening of the larynx, the opening is guarded by a flap of tissue called *epiglottis.* The most important structures of the larynx are the *vocal folds,* sometimes called *vocal cords,* which act like musical strings and are set in vibration by the passage of air. The vibration produces the sound.

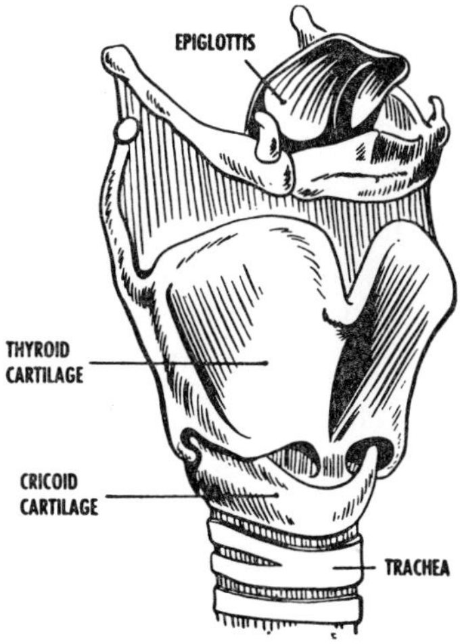

Figure 112. Front view of the cartilages of the larynx.

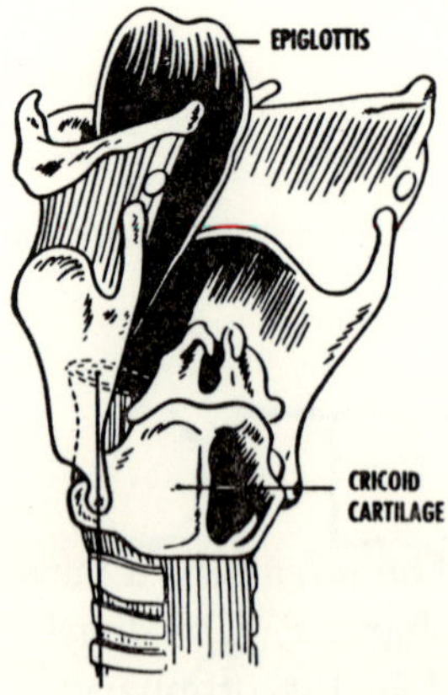

Figure 113. Posterior view of the larynx.

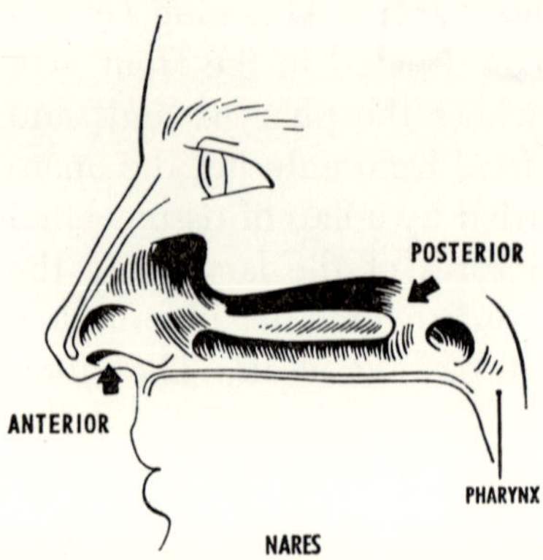

Figure 114. Sagittal section through nasal passages showing anterior and posterior nares.

The Trachea and the Bronchi: The air which travels down the pharynx enters the *trachea* or windpipe through the larynx, which sits on the top of the trachea. The trachea is a tubular structure which extends into the chest cavity behind the heart. At its lower end it divides into two branches, a *left bronchus* and a *right bronchus* (plural, *bronchi*). Each bronchus enters its corresponding lung at an indented place called *hilus* (sometimes *hilum*). In the lung the bronchus divides into smaller and smaller branches, the *bronchioles,* which terminate in microscopic sacs, the *alveoli* (singular, *alveolus*). The exchange of oxygen and carbon dioxide between the blood and the lung tissue takes place at the alveoli. Collectively, the bronchi and their branches are known as the *bronchial tree,* because of the natural resemblance.

The Lungs: Each lung, composed of bronchial tubes, alveoli, blood vessels and nerves, is a cone-shaped organ so placed in the chest that its *apex* points upward and its *base* is in contact with the surface of the diaphragm. The lungs are surrounded by a double-layered sac, the *pleura.* The space between the lungs is the *mediastinum.* It contains the heart, the great blood vessels, the esophagus, and part of the trachea. The right lung is divided by two *interlobar fissures* into three lobes: the *superior lobe,* the *middle lobe,* and *inferior lobe.* The left lung is divided into two lobes: the superior and inferior. The layer of the pleura which covers the lung is the *visceral pleura.* The other layer, which lines the inner surface of the chest wall, is the *parietal pleura.* Inflammation of the pleura is *pleuritis.* The blood vessels and bronchi which leave or enter the lung at the hilus are known collectively as the *root of the lung.*

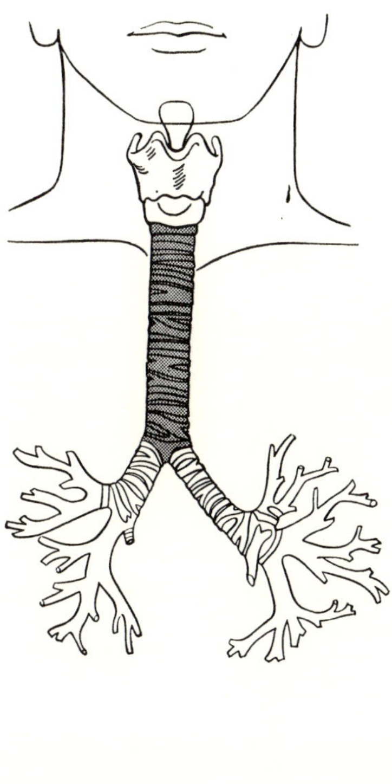

Figure 115. The larynx, trachea, and the bronchial tree.

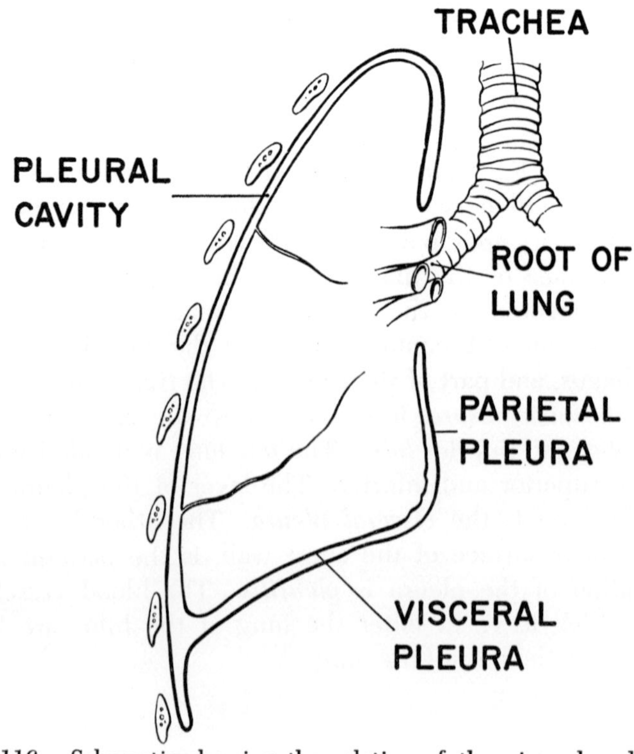

Figure 116. Schematic showing the relation of the visceral and parietal layers of the pleura.

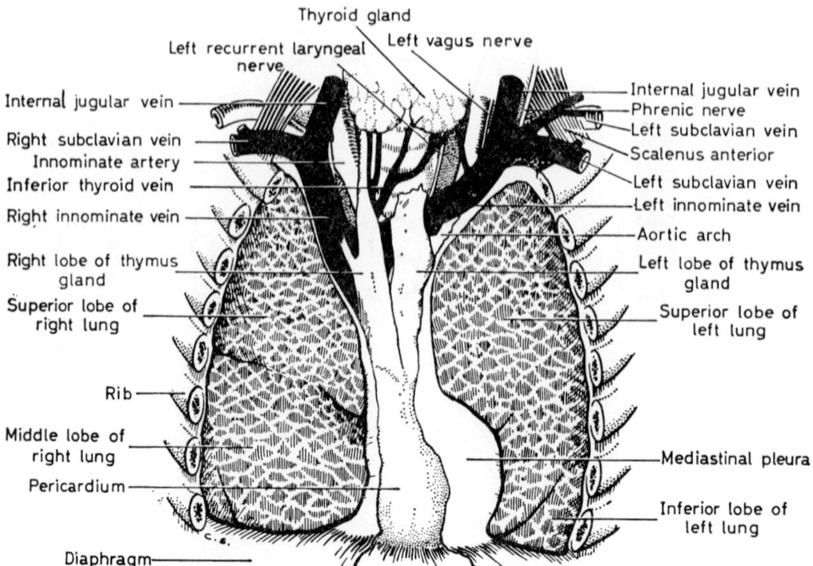

Figure 117. Detailed study of the structures of the thoracic cavity.

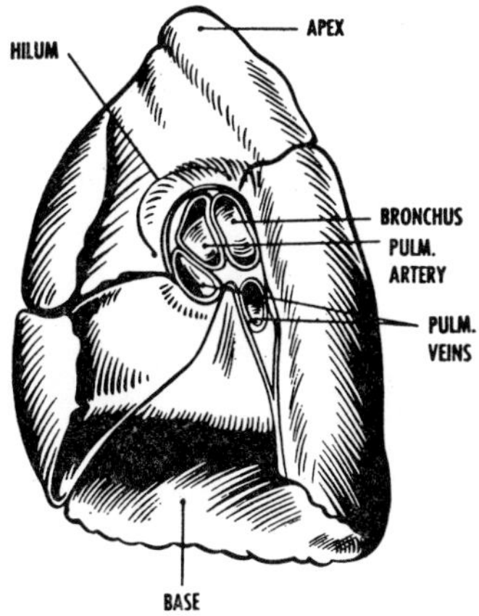

Figure 118. The medial aspect of the lung, showing the bronchus and the great blood vessels.

VOCABULARY REVIEW

Define the following terms on the basis of the preceding discussion. Consult a medical dictionary for the correct pronunciation.

adenoids
alveoli
alveolus
apex
base
bronchi
bronchial tree
bronchiole
bronchus
carbon dioxide
choanae
cilia
epiglottis
expiration
hilum
hilus
inferior lobe
inspiration
interlobar fissure
larynx
left bronchus
lung
mediastinum
middle lobe
nasopharynx
oropharynx
oxygen
parietal pleura
pleura
pleuritis
posterior nares
respiration
right bronchus
root of lung
superior lobe
tonsils
trachea
vibrissae
visceral pleura
vocal cords
vocal folds

REVIEW QUESTIONS

1. What are the medical terms for *breathing in* and *breathing out?*
2. What are the *hair-like projections* on the mucous membrane called?
3. What do you call the *upper portion* of the pharynx?
4. What are the back openings of the nose called?
5. What is the common name of the larynx?
6. What is the medical term for *windpipe?*
7. What do you call the "musical strings" that produce the voice?
8. What are the divisions of the trachea called?
9. What are the branches of the trachea called?
10. What is the space between the lungs called?
11. Into what is the lung anatomically divided?
12. What is meant by the root of the lung?

Chapter XI

THE URINARY SYSTEM

GENERAL CONSIDERATIONS. Some of the waste products of metabolism present in the blood are removed in the process of breathing, but it remains for the urinary system to remove the soluble, nonvolatile matter. This is accomplished by a complex method of filtration that takes place in the kidneys, where the blood is brought into close contact with a system of tubes that absorb the waste through a thin layer of cells (which acts in the manner of a chemical filter paper). The gross structures of the urinary system are the *kidneys*, the *ureters*, the *bladder*, and the *urethra*.

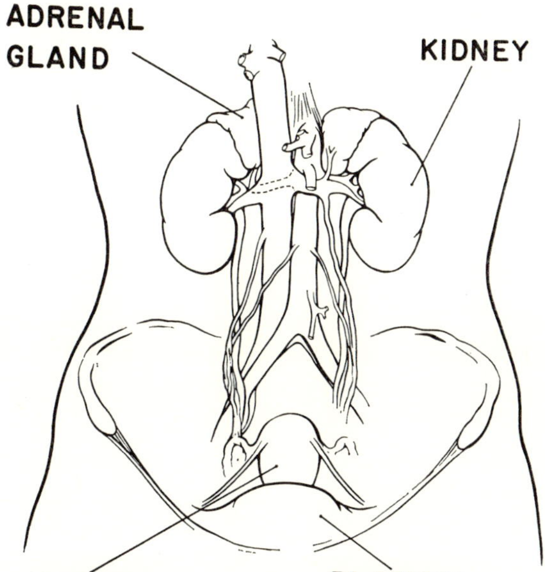

Figure 119. Urinary organs of the female.

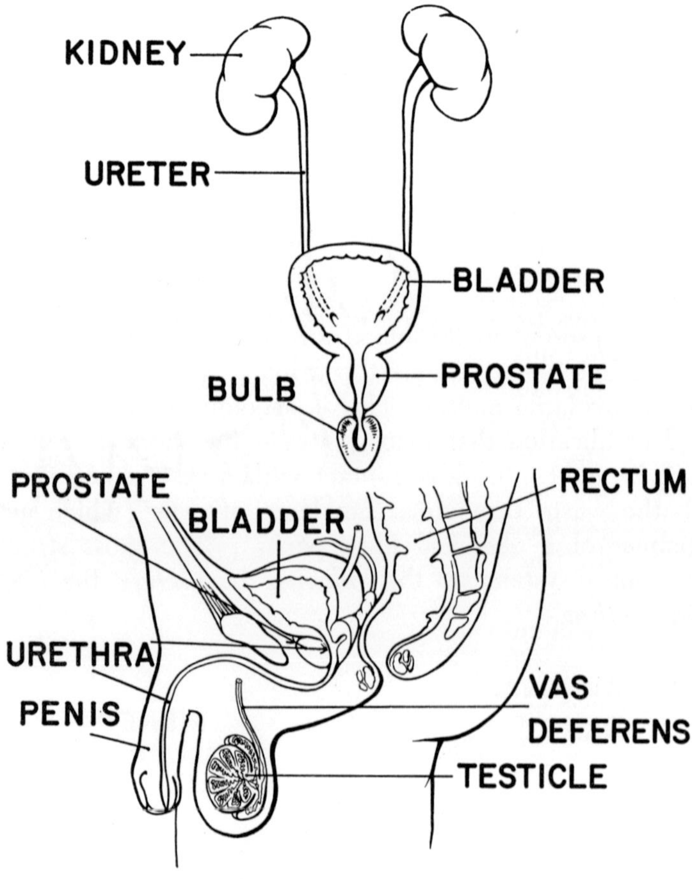

Figure 120. Front and side views of the male urinary organs.

The Kidneys: There are two kidneys, one on each side of the vertebral column. Each kidney is embedded in fatty tissue and is surrounded by a tough membrane, the *capsule*. The medial border of the kidney has a notch, the *hilus* or *hilum,* where connections are made with the blood vessels and a slender tube, the *ureter*. The ureter, which may be envisioned as an elongated stem of a funnel, expands in the kidney to form the *renal pelvis* (which is similar to the upper, expanded portion of a funnel). The pelvis receives urine from smaller funnel-like structures, the *calices* (singular, *calyx*). The calices receive the urine from tiny "faucets" called *papillae,* which collect the urine from *collecting tubules.* A collecting tubule is the terminal part of the delicate filtering unit of the kidney, the *nephron.*

The Nephron: This is the structure which removes the waste-laden fluid from the blood and converts it into urine. The action begins in the *renal corpuscle,* a microscopic structure where a tiny tuft of blood vessels, the *glomerulus,* is lodged in an invagination of the blind beginning of a tube, *Bowman's capsule.* The fluid passes from the tuft into the tube at this point. The tube or *tubule* (small tube) continues for a considerable distance within the substance of the kidney. It is divided into three segments: the *proximal convoluted tubule, Henle's loop* (which has a *descending limb* and *ascending limb*), and the *distal convoluted tubule.* As the fluid passes through the segments of the tubule, some of the water and certain constituents are reabsorbed by the blood. The resulting fluid is the *urine.* The distal convoluted tubule finally discharges the urine into the collecting tubule, which in turn discharges it into a calyx and the pelvis of the kidney.

The Ureter: The pelvis of the kidney may be regarded as the

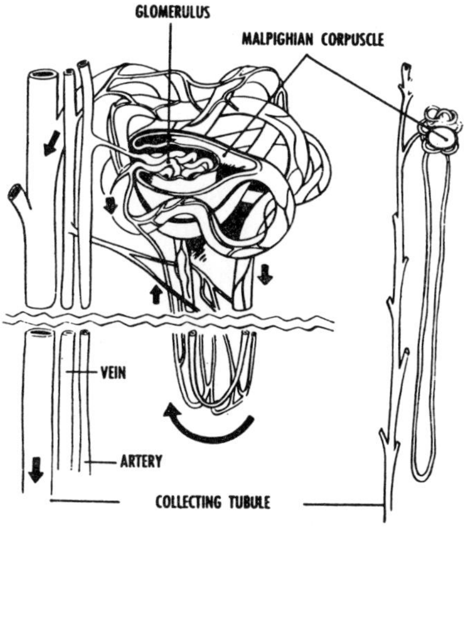

Figure 121. Microscopic structure of a nephron, the structural unit of the kidney.

expanded upper end of the *ureter,* the slender tube which carries the urine from the kidney to the bladder. There is one ureter for each kidney.

The Urinary Bladder: This structure is a muscular sac in which the urine is temporarily stored. The *urinary bladder* has three openings on its floor. Two of the openings admit the urine from the ureters. The third is the outlet of the bladder, which leads to the *urethra.* The three openings mark a triangular area, the *trigone* of the urinary bladder.

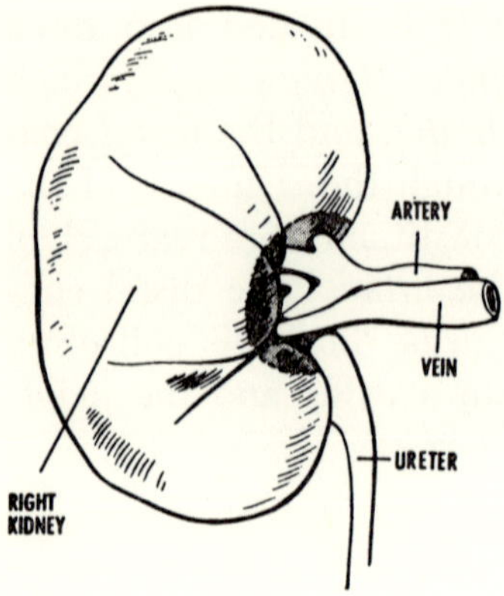

Figure 122. The hilus of the kidney, showing the ureter and the blood vessels.

The Urethra: The urine is discharged from the urinary bladder through a channel called the *urethra.* The male urethra, which is longer than the female, is divided into three portions: the *prostatic urethra* (which is the nearest to the bladder), the *membranous urethra,* and the *cavernous urethra.* The latter extends through the *penis,* the male copulative organ.

Formation and Discharge: The urine begins to form in the renal corpuscle, where fluid containing dissolved waste passes from the glomerulus into the capsule of Bowman. The fluid then travels through the proximal convoluted tubule, Henle's loop, the distal convoluted tubule, and the collecting tubule. From here the urine passes into a calyx, the pelvis of the kidney, a ureter, the bladder, and the urethra, which discharges it to the

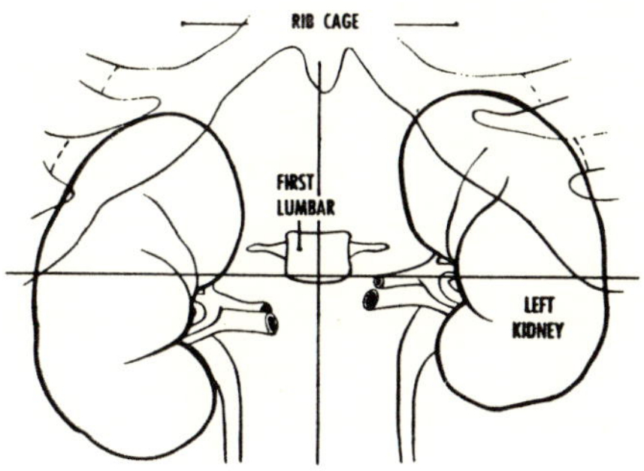

Figure 123. Diagram of the kidneys, showing relation to the level of the ribs and vertebrae.

outside. The discharge of urine is called *micturition* or *voiding*. Involuntary micturition is called *incontinence*. The urine is kept within the bladder by an *external sphincter* and an *internal sphincter*, which control the passage into and out of the urethra. When the sphincters are contracted, the urine remains in the bladder. Relaxation of the sphincters permits the discharge.

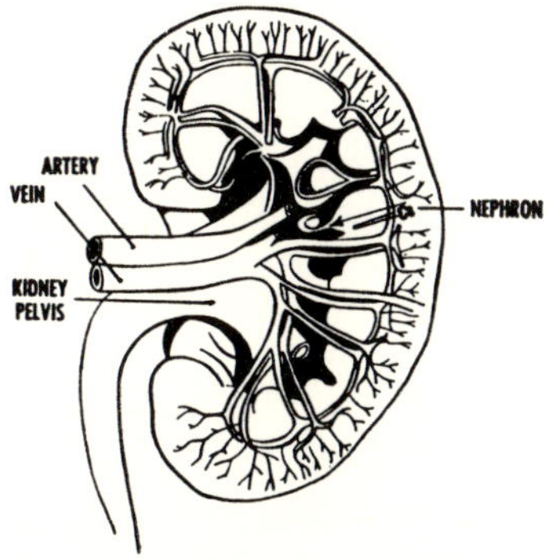

Figure 124. Sagittal section of the kidney.

VOCABULARY REVIEW

Define the following terms on the basis of the preceding discussion. Consult a medical dictionary for the correct pronunciation.

ascending limb
bladder
Bowman's capsule
calices
calyx
capsule
cavernous urethra
collecting tubule
descending limb
distal convoluted tubule
external sphincter
glomerulus
Henle's loop
hilus
incontinence
internal sphincter
kidney
membranous urethra
micturition
nephron
papillae
penis
prostatic urethra
proximal convoluted tubule
renal corpuscle
renal pelvis
trigone
tubule
ureter
urethra
urinary bladder
urine
voiding

REVIEW QUESTIONS

1. What is the difference between the *urethra* and a *ureter*?
2. What is meant by a *renal pelvis*?
3. What is a *calyx* and what is the plural form of this term?
4. What is a *nephron*? How does it compare with a *neuron*?
5. What does a *glomerulus* consist of? What is *Bowman's capsule*?
6. In what structure do you find a *descending limb*?
7. What is the *trigone* and how many openings does it have?
8. Into how many parts is the *urethra* divided?
9. What is the medical term for discharging the urine?
10. The involuntary discharge of urine is called what?

Chapter XII

THE REPRODUCTIVE SYSTEM

GENERAL CONSIDERATIONS. The purpose of the reproductive system in the male and in the female is to provide the necessary cells from the union of which a new organism may develop. The reproductive systems begin to function at the age of puberty, about age 12 in girls and 14 in boys. At this time the *secondary sex characteristics* begin to appear as a result of the hormonal activity of the sex glands. In the male, the sex characteristics begin to show in the growth of a beard, *pubic hair* (hair around the penis), and *axillary hair* (hair in the armpits). There is also a change in voice to the deeper tones. In the female, the breasts begin to develop at this time and there is also a growth of pubic and axillary hair. The most outstanding change, however, is the appearance of *menstruation.* The chief male hormone is *testosterone;* the female hormones are *estrogen* and *progesterone.*

MALE REPRODUCTIVE SYSTEM: The chief structures of this system are the *testes,* the *excretory ducts,* the *auxiliary glands,* and the *penis.*

The Testes: The *testes* (singular, *testis*) or *testicles* are egg-shaped structures situated in the *scrotum* (a fleshy sac) below the penis. Each testicle is surrounded by a *capsule* and is divided into *lobules.* The lobules contain *seminiferous tubules,* where the reproductive cells are formed. The tubules unite to form *efferent ducts* which lead to the *epididymis,* a mass of ducts situated on the top of the testicle. These ducts terminate in a larger duct, the *ductus epididymis,* which in turn becomes the *ductus deferens.* The ductus deferens enters the abdomen (through the *external inguinal ring* and the *internal inguinal ring*) and (along with a duct from the *seminal vesicle*) joins the *urethra,* which leads to the outside.

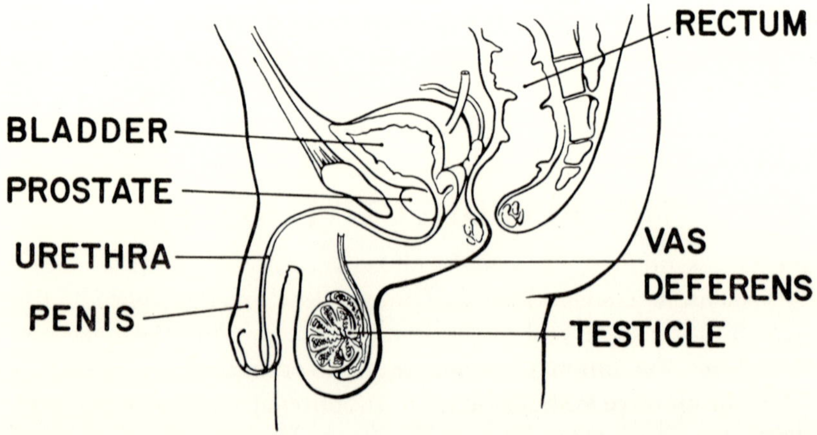

Figure 125. Sagittal section or side view of the male reproductive organs.

The function of the testis is twofold: to produce *spermatozoa* (singular, *spermatozoon*), also known as *sperm, germ cells,* and *reproductive cells;* and to produce male hormones, especially *testosterone.*

The Spermatozoa: The male reproductive cells are produced in the seminiferous tubules of the testis, specifically by the *spermatogenic* or *germinal* cells. The germinal cells produce the *spermatogonium,* the earliest form of the spermatozoon. The spermatogonium matures into a *spermatocyte,* which develops into a *spermatid.* The spermatid finally forms the functional spermatozoon. The mature spermatozoa enter the seminiferous tubules and follow the ducts described above. They are ejected through the penis during *ejaculation* (the ejection of the semen during the male orgasm).

The Male Hormones: Between the seminiferous tubules, the testis contains an *interstitial tissue* composed of *epithelioid* cells. This tissue contains the so-called *Leydig cells,* which are believed to produce the *androgens* (the male sex hormones). The production of the androgens in the testis is under the control of *gonadotropic hormones* of the *pituitary gland,* which is located below the brain.

Epididymis: This structure, lying along the upper and

posterior surface of the testis, is composed mainly of the convoluted portion of the excretory duct of the testis between the efferent ducts and the ducus deferens (described above).

Ductus Deferens: The ductus deferens is the continuation of the epididymis. It enters the abdomen to unite with the duct of the seminal vesicle, thus forming the *ejaculatory duct*.

Ejaculatory Duct: This short, straight tube penetrates the prostate gland and opens into the urethra.

Spermatic Cord: The *spermatic cord* is composed of the ductus deferens, blood vessels, and nerves. It begins at the testicle and extends into the abdomen.

Seminal Vesicles: The seminal vesicle, one on each side, is a pouch-like structure which produces some of the fluid in which the spermatozoa are carried. Its duct joins the ductus deferens to form the ejaculatory duct.

The Penis: The copulative organ of the male is composed of three cylindrical shafts of *erectile tissue*. Two of these, the *corpora cavernosa penis*, are situated side by side and form the dorsal part of the penis. The third shaft, the *corpus cavernosum urethrae*, lies in the groove between and below the other two. The three shafts are surrounded and covered by fascia and skin. The erectile tissue of the penis has cavern-like spaces which fill with blood during sexual excitement, changing the organ to a

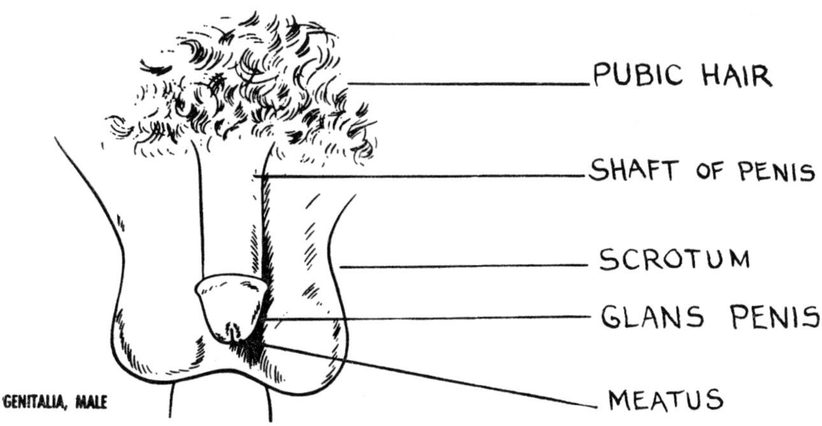

Figure 126. The male genital organ.

rigid and erect form. The cone-shaped head of the penis, the *glans penis,* is an expansion of the corpus cavernosum urethrae. A hood-like layer of skin covers the glans. It is known as the *prepuce* or *foreskin.* The surgical removal of the prepuce is *circumcision.*

The Semen: The *semen* or *seminal fluid,* which is ejected from the penis during the acme of copulation, is composed of a fluid (formed in the ducts and auxiliary glands) and the reproductive cells, or spermatozoa.

VOCABULARY REVIEW

Define the following terms on the basis of the preceding discussion. Determine the pronunciation by consulting a medical dictionary.

androgens
auxiliary glands
axillary hair
capsule
circumcision
corpora cavernosa penis
corpus cavernosum urethrae
ductus deferens
ductus epididymis
efferent ducts
ejaculation
ejaculatory duct
epididymis
epithelioid cells
erectile tissue
estrogen
excretory ducts
external inguinal ring
foreskin
germ cells
germinal cells
glans penis
gonadotropic hormone
internal inguinal ring
interstitial tissue
Leydig cells
lobule
penis
pituitary gland
prepuce
progesterone
pubic hair
reproductive cells
scrotum
secondary sex characteristics
semen
seminal fluid
seminal vesicle
seminiferous tubules
sperm
spermatic cord
spermatid
spermatocyte
spermatogenic cells
spermatogonium
spermatozoa
spermatozoon
testes
testicle
testis
testosterone
urethra

Female Reproductive System. The female reproductive organs are the *ovaries, uterine tubes, uterus, vagina, external genitalia,* and the *breasts.*

The Ovaries: The ovaries, which correspond to the testes of the male, produce the *ova* (singular, *ovum*), the female reproductive cells. They are situated in the pelvis (lower part of the abdomen). The central portion of the ovary is the *medulla;* the outer portion is the *cortex.* The cortex, with *germinal epithelium,* contains *graafian follicles* (where the ova are developed). The discharge of an ovum from the ovary is called

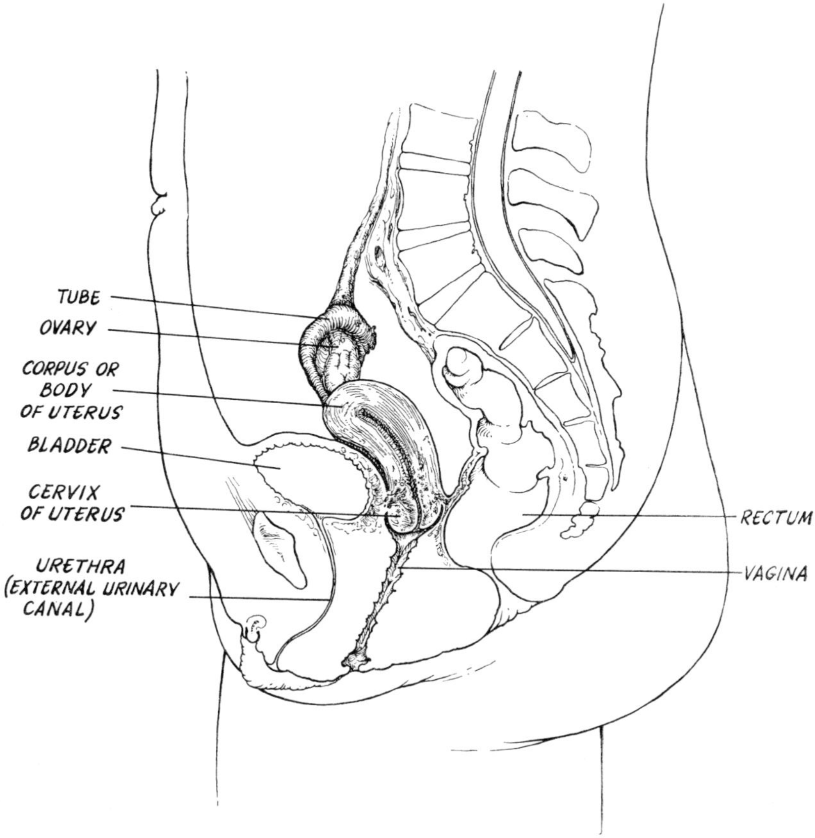

Figure 127. Diagrammatic side view of the female reproductive organs.

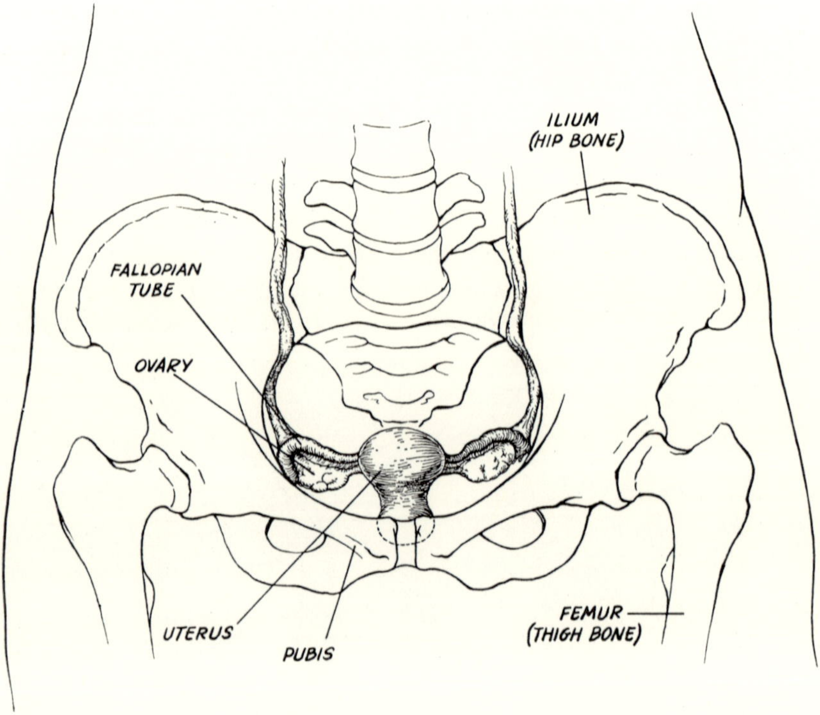

Figure 128. Front view of the female pelvic structures and the ovaries.

ovulation. After the discharge of an ovum, the graafian follicle which contained it becomes the *corpus luteum.*

Uterine Tubes: These tubes or ducts are also called *fallopian tubes.* There is one on each side of the *uterus* or womb. One end is attached to and opens into the uterus; the other end remains open and is situated at the side of the pelvis. The tube, which is about 12 cm in length, is placed horizontally and lies within a fold of peritoneum, the *broad ligament.* The lateral end of the *uterine tube* widens into a funnel-shaped pouch called *infundibulum,* which has finger-like projections called *fimbriae.*

The Uterus: The uterus or womb is a hollow, pear-shaped organ within which the fertilized ovum develops into an *embryo* and *fetus.* (During the first two months, the product of pregnancy is called embryo; after that, fetus.) The pear-shaped

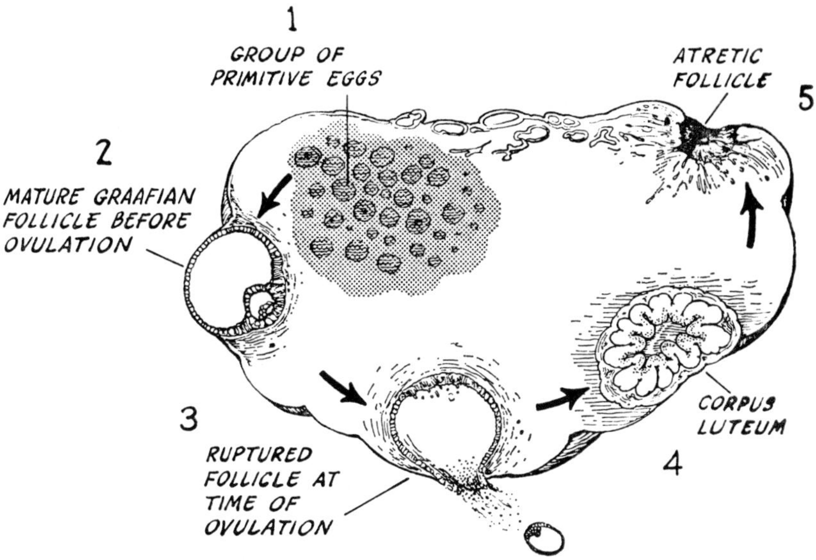

Figure 129. Diagrammatic sketch of the ovary, showing structures associated with the menstrual cycle.

uterus is situated in the pelvis, between the bladder and the rectum, with its tapering end downward. The larger upper portion of the organ is the *body*. The lower, tapering end is the *cervix* (which protrudes into the upper part of the vagina). The rounded upper part of the body of the uterus, above the entrance of the uterine tubes, is the *fundus*. The wall of the uterus is composed of three layers of tissue: the innermost, the *endometrium*, is made of mucous membrane; the middle layer, the *myometrium*, is composed of smooth muscle; the outer layer is composed of peritoneum or serous membrane.

The Vagina: The vagina is a muscular tube which extends from the cervix of the uterus above to the opening below between the anus and the urethra. It is thus situated between the bladder and urethra (in front) and the rectum (in the back). Where the cervix projects into the vagina, there is a circular recess called *fornix*. The mucous membrane lining the vagina lies in transverse folds, the *vaginal rugae*. The outlet or opening of the

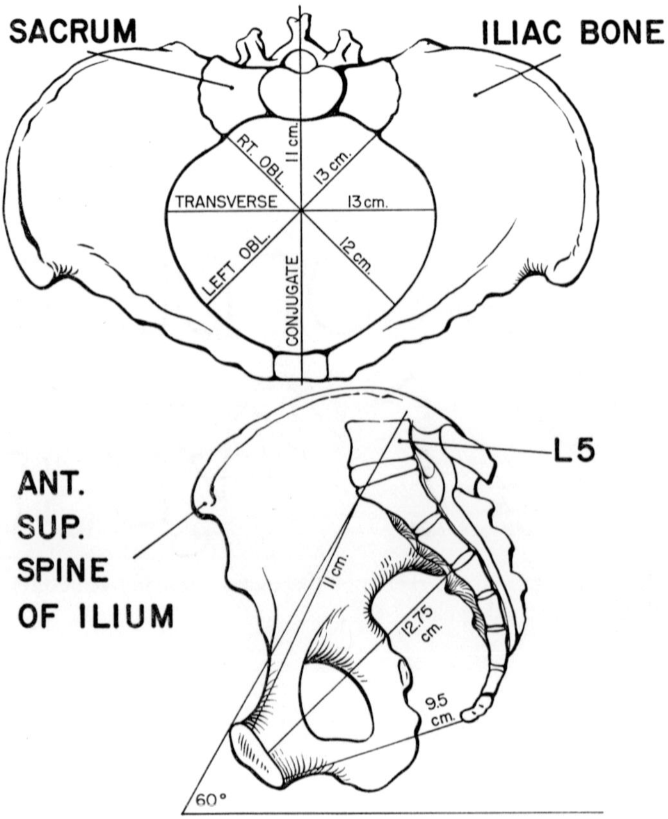

Figure 130. Measurements of the female pelvis.

vagina (between the urethra and anus) is partially covered by a fold of mucous membrane, the *hymen.*

External Genitalia: The structures concerned with reproduction that are situated at or near the surface of the body (between the thighs) are known collectively as the *external genitalia, external genital organs,* and *vulva.* These structures are the *mons pubis,* the *labia majora,* the *labia minora,* the *clitoris,* and the *vestibule.* The mons pubis is formed by a pad of fatty tissue at the junction of the pubic bones, just above the cleft. It is covered with pubic hair after puberty. The labia majora (singular, *labium majus*) are two folds of connective tissue covered with

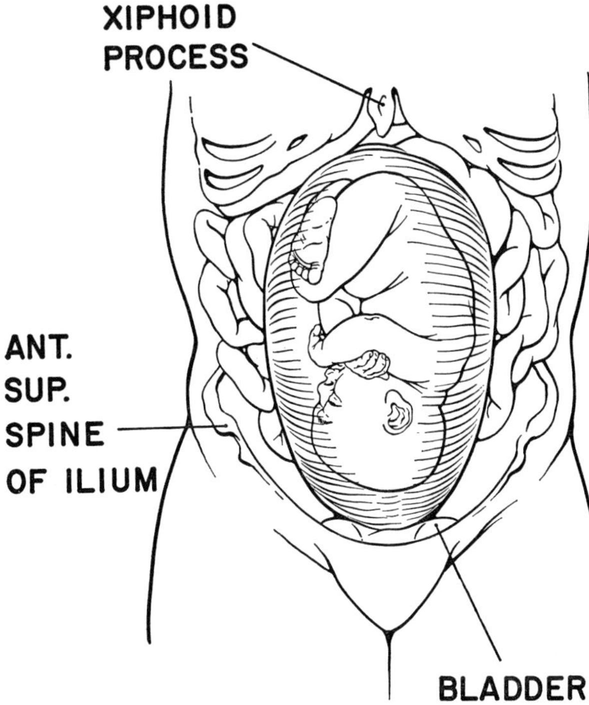

Figure 131. Sketch of pregnant uterus, showing position of fetus.

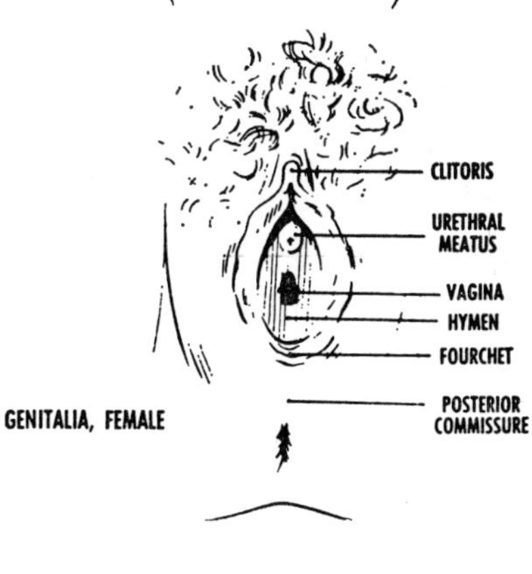

Figure 132. The external reproductive organs of the female.

skin, one on each side, between the inner surface of the thigh and the cleft. They almost completely disappear when the thighs are abducted. Between the labia majora are two similar structures of smaller size, the *labia minora.* They are covered by mucous membrane. The region between the labia minora (singular, *labium minus*) is called the *vestibule.* It contains the *vaginal orifice* and the *urethral orifice,* i.e. the openings of the

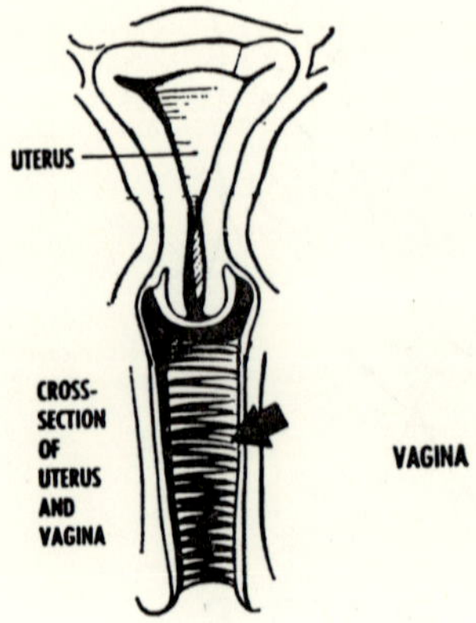

Figure 133. Sketch showing relation of uterus to vagina.

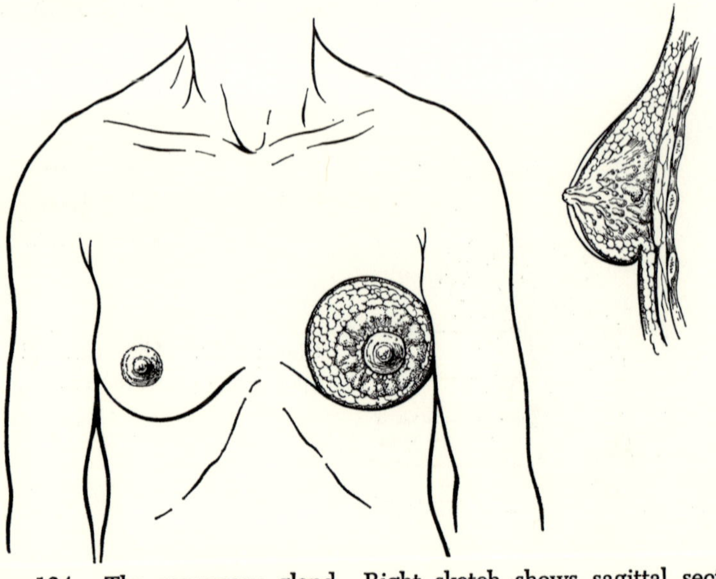

Figure 134. The mammary gland. Right sketch shows sagittal section.

vagina and the urethra. The clitoris, a small penis-like structure, is situated at the junction of the labia minora in front.

The breasts or *mammary glands* are regarded as accessory organs of the reproductive system. Each breast is divided into 15 to 25 lobes, which are the glands that produce the milk. The duct of each lobe or gland extends toward the nipple or *mammilla.* The individual glands and their ducts thus form a radiating structure similar to the spokes of a wheel, with the nipple forming the hub. Each duct opens through the nipple. The pigmented circle around the nipple is the *areola.*

The Perineum: The term *perineum* may be applied to the region at the lower end of the trunk between the symphysis pubis in front and the sacrum in the back. In the female, it contains all of the structures described above. Some clinicians limit the term to the region between the opening of the vagina and the anus.

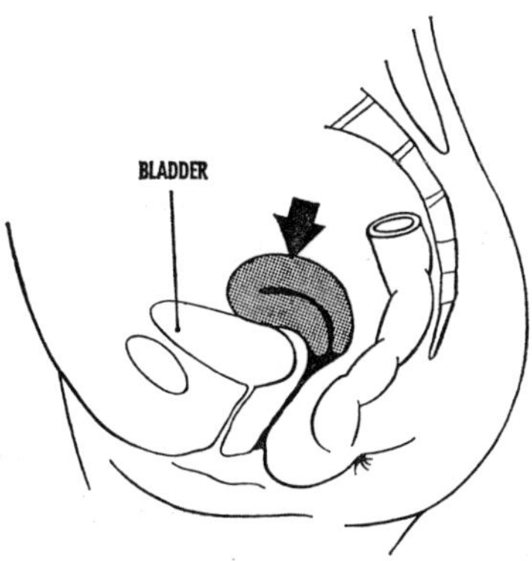

Figure 135. Side view of the normal position of the uterus.

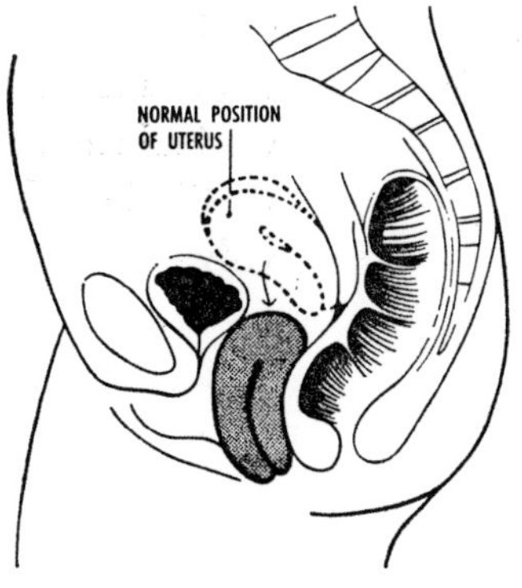

Figure 136. Abnormal displacement of the uterus downward.

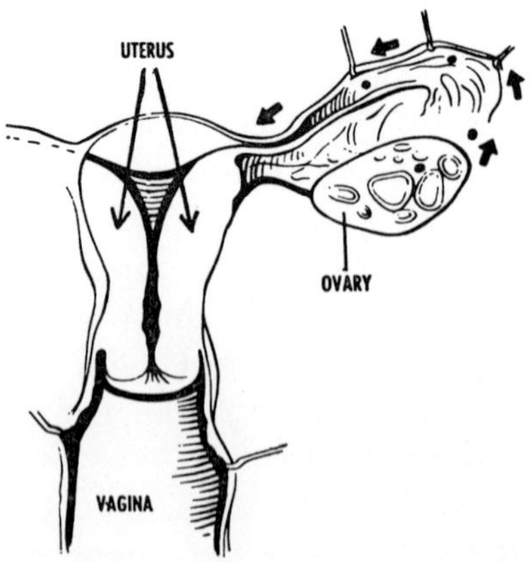

Figure 137. Sketch showing migration of the ovum from the ovary to the uterus through the uterine tube.

VOCABULARY REVIEW

Define the following terms on the basis of the preceding discussion. Determine the pronunciation with the aid of a medical dictionary.

areola	fimbriae	myometrium
body	fornix	ova
breast	fundus	ovaries
broad ligament	germinal epithelium	ovary
cervix	graafian follicles	ovulation
clitoris	hymen	ovum
corpus luteum	infundibulum	perineum
cortex	labia majora	urethral orifice
embryo	labia minora	uterine tubes
endometrium	labium majus	uterus
external genital organs	labium minus	vagina
	mammary glands	vaginal orifice
external genitalia	mammilla	vaginal rugae
fallopian tube	medulla	vestibule
fetus	mons pubis	vulva

REVIEW EXERCISES

1. What is meant by secondary sex characteristics? What are they?
2. Name the principal male hormone and two female hormones.
3. What is the plural form of *testis*?
4. Where would you find *seminiferous tubules*?
5. What is meant by *epididymis,* and what is the plural form?
6. What are the principal functions of the testes?
7. What are the *spermatozoa,* and what is the singular form?
8. What are *spermatogenic* or *germinal* cells? Where are they found?
9. What is a *spermatogonium,* and what is the plural of this term?
10. What are *epithelioid cells*? Look up the etymology of *epithelioid.*
11. What are the combining forms of the word *androgen*?
12. Where are the *Leydig cells* to be found?
13. Which of the endocrine glands produces *gonadotropic* hormones?
14. Check the component parts of *gonadotropic.*
15. Name the three shafts of erectile tissue forming the penis.
16. What is the *corpus cavernousm urethrae*?
17. Give the medical term for *foreskin.*
18. Name the reproductive organs of the female.
19. What is an *ovum*? What is the plural?
20. What is a *graafian follicle*? What is the derivation of the term?
21. What is meant by *ovulation*? Where do you find the *corpus luteum*?
22. Where are the *fallopian tubes* located? What are the *uterine tubes*?
23. What is the difference between an *embryo* and a *fetus*?
24. What is the cervix of the uterus?
25., Name the *lining membrane* and the *muscular layer* of the uterus.

Chapter XIII

THE AUDITORY SYSTEM

HEARING AND EQUILIBRIUM. The ear is concerned with the functions of *hearing* and *equilibrium*. The ear is divided into three parts: the *external ear*, the *middle ear*, and the *inner ear*. All three parts are concerned with hearing; only the inner ear is concerned with equilibrium.

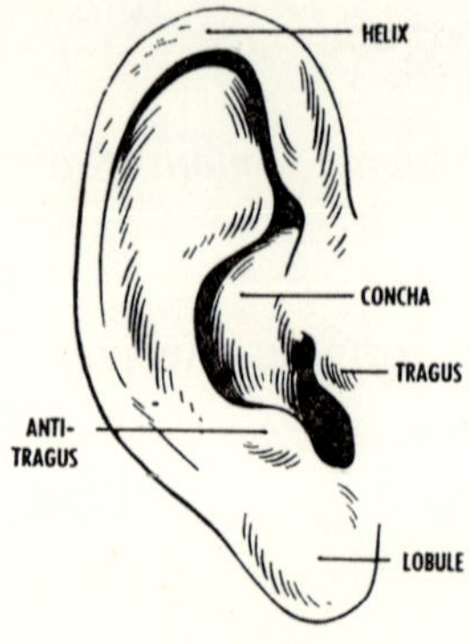

Figure 138. The named components of the auricle or pinna.

External Ear: This consists of the *pinna* or *auricle* (the part projecting from the side of the head) and the *external acoustic meatus*, the canal or passage which extends from the outer opening of the ear to the eardrum, also known as the *auditory canal*. The lining of this passage secretes a waxy substance called *cerumen*.

Middle Ear: The middle ear is a small chamber separated from the external ear by the eardrum or *tympanum*. Within the middle ear are three *ossicles* or little bones: the *malleus* (hammer), *incus* (anvil), and *stapes* (stirrup). The sound or vibrating air enters the ear through the external acoustic meatus and causes the tympanum to vibrate. The vibration is transmitted to the inner ear through the ossicles. The middle ear communicates with the pharynx by means of a tube, the *eustachian* or *auditory tube.*

Inner Ear: This is the most complex of the three parts. It contains the organs for hearing and equilibrium. It is also known as the *labyrinth.* Its bony part is called *osseous labyrinth;* the membranous part is the *membranous labyrinth.* The membranous part lies within the bony part and is separated from it by a fluid called *perilymph.* The fluid within the membranous part is called *endolymph.* The inner ear is composed of three structures: the *cochlea* (in front), the *vestibule* (in the middle), and the *semicircular canals* (behind). The vestibule and semicircular

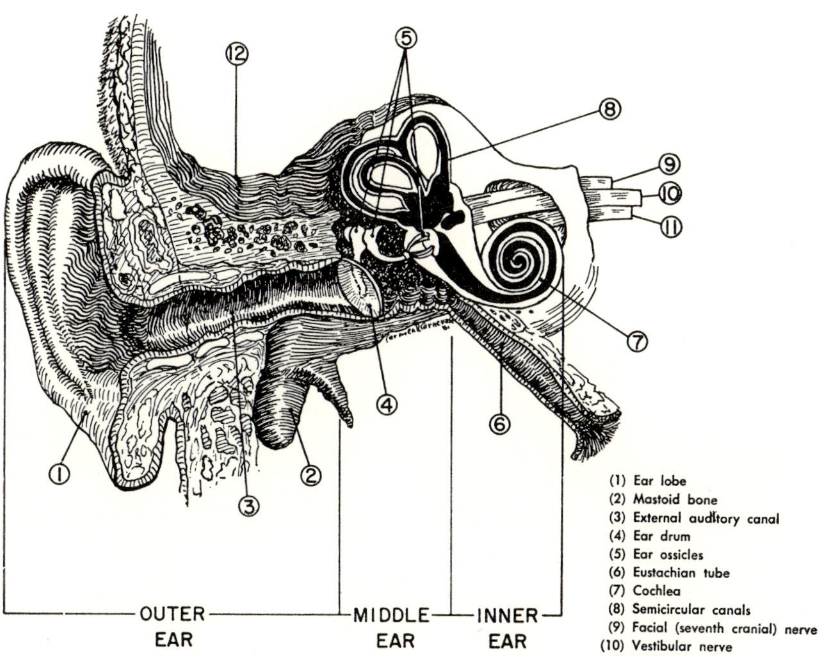

Figure 139. A frontal section through the structures of the ear, showing the principal divisions and component parts.

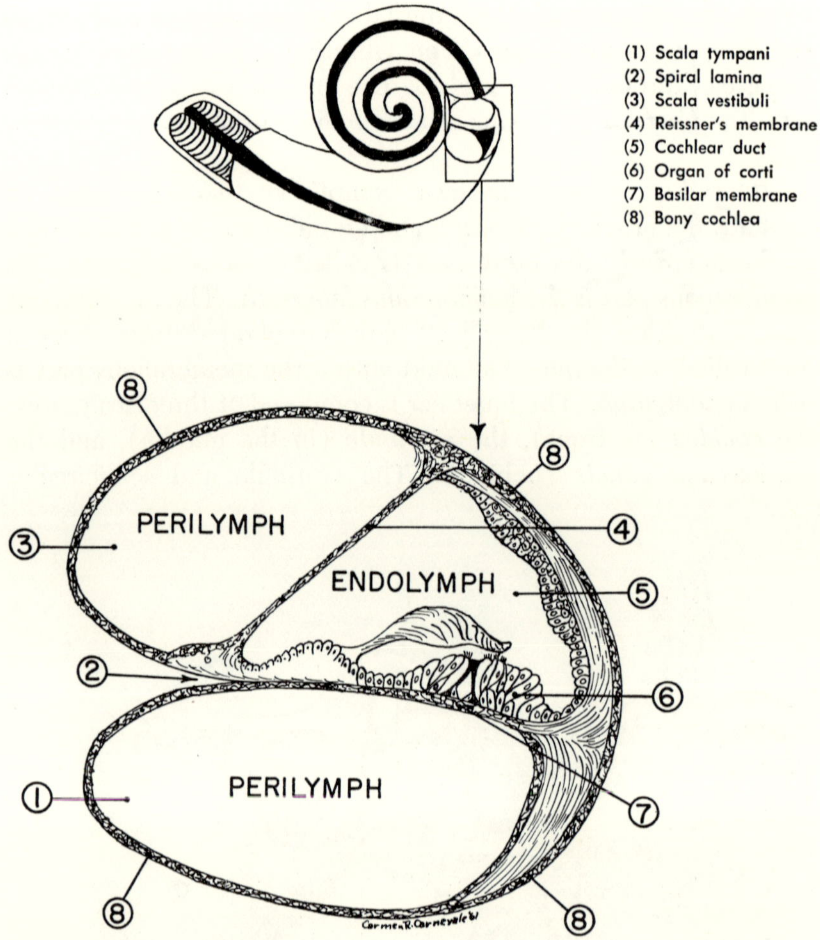

Figure 140. A cross-section of the cochlea of the inner ear, where sound vibrations are transformed into nerve impulses.

canals are concerned with equilibrium, the cochlea with hearing.

The Vestibule: This structure contains the *saccule* and *utricle*, which along with the semicircular canals contain the mechanism for the senses of position and movement of the head (and hence equilibrium). Each ear has three semicircular canals placed at right angles to one another. They are the *posterior, superior,* and *lateral semicircular canals.*

The Cochlea: The cochlea resembles the shell of a snail and is basically a twisted tube divided into an upper and a lower passageway. The upper passage is the *scala vestibuli*. The lower passage is the *scala tympani*. The scala vestibuli ends at the *fenestra vestibuli* or *oval window*, while the scala tympani ends at the *fenestra cochleae* or *round window*. The fenestra vestibuli receives vibrations from the stapes (mentioned above). The nerve impulses generated in the inner ear are transmitted to the brain by the *vestibulocochlear nerve* (also known as *acoustic nerve* and *auditory nerve*).

VOCABULARY REVIEW

Define the following terms on the basis of the preceding discussion. Determine the pronunciation with the aid of a medical dictionary.

- acoustic nerve
- anvil
- auditory
- auditory canal
- auditory nerve
- auditory tube
- auricle
- cerumen
- cochlea
- endolymph
- equilibrium
- eustachian tube
- external acoustic meatus
- external ear
- fenestra cochleae
- fenestra vestibuli
- hammer
- incus
- inner ear
- labyrinth
- lateral semicircular canal
- malleus
- membranous labyrinth
- middle ear
- osseous labyrinth
- ossicles
- oval window
- perilymph
- pinna
- posterior semicircular canal
- round window
- saccule
- scala tympani
- scala vestibuli
- semicircular canals
- stapes
- stirrup
- superior semicircular canal
- tympanum
- utricle
- vestibule
- vestibulocochlear nerve

REVIEW EXERCISES

1. Name the three divisions of the ear.
2. What is the function of the *external acoustic meatus*?
3. The waxy substance formed in the external ear is called what?
4. Name the three small bones of the middle ear.
5. What is the medical term for the *eardrum*?
6. What is a synonym for a *eustachian tube*?
7. What is the technical medical term for the *inner ear*?
8. Name the three principal structures of the inner ear.
9. What is the function of the semicircular canals?
10. What two structures are found in the vestibule of the ear?
11. What nerve transmits the impulses from the inner ear to the brain?

Chapter XIV

THE VISUAL SYSTEM

GENERAL CONSIDERATIONS. The visual apparatus is composed of the eyeball and its supporting and auxiliary structures, the optic nerve, and the cortex of the brain. The light coming from a particular object enters the eye and stimulates certain nerve structures. The generated impulses are conveyed by the optic nerve to the cortex of the occipital lobe of the brain.

The Eyeball: The eyeball is spherical in shape and is situated in the *orbit* or *eye socket*. Its walls are composed of three layers: the outer *sclera*, the middle *choroid*, and the inner *retina*. The sclera is a tough fibrous coat which is modified in front to form the transparent *cornea*. The choroid has many blood vessels and is concerned with the nutrition of the eye. The front part of the choroid is modified in structure and is known as the *ciliary body* (composed of the *ciliary muscle* and *ciliary process*), which supports the *crystalline lens*.

The ciliary body also supports the *iris*, the pigmented circular structure with its central *pupil*, situated behind the cornea and in front of the lens. The retina is the inner coat or lining of the eyeball. It is a nerve structure continuous with the *optic nerve*, which carries the stimuli to the brain. The place where the optic nerve leaves the eyeball is called the *optic disk*, which is also the *blind spot*. Near the center of the back of the eye, on the inside, is a yellowish spot, the *macula lutea*. In the center of this is the *fovea centralis*, a small depression. It is the region of sharpest vision. The space within the eyeball in front of the iris is the *anterior chamber*. The space between the iris and the lens is the *posterior chamber*. The space between the cornea and the lens is filled with a fluid called *aqueous humor*. The space behind the lens is filled with a viscid substance called *vitreous humor*.

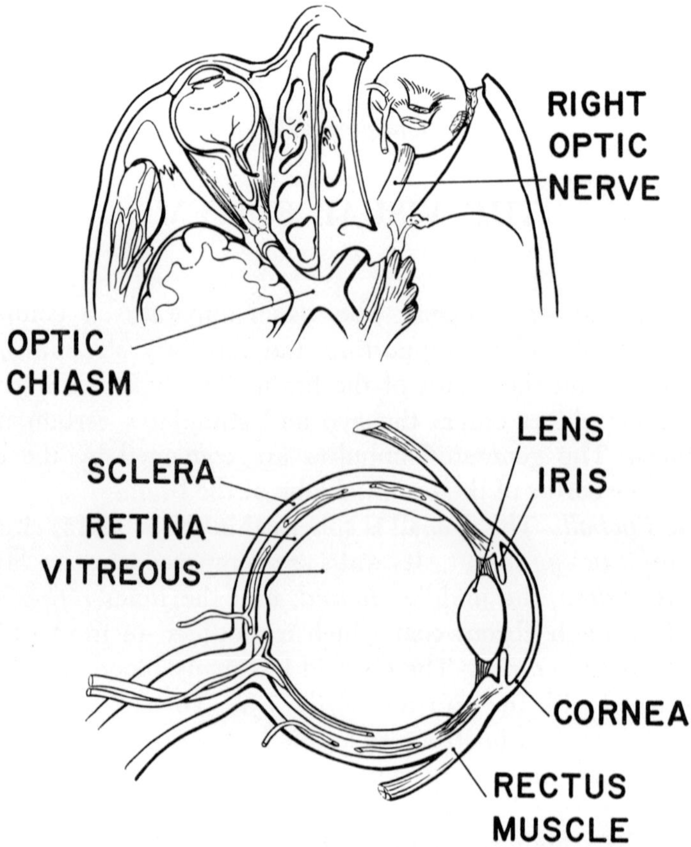

Figure 141. Upper illustration shows a transverse section of the skull at the level of the eyes. Note the course of the optic nerve. Lower sketch shows a simplified sagittal section of the eye. The vascular layer between the sclera and the retina is the choroid.

Auxiliary Structures: The eyeball is covered by a transparent membrane, the *conjunctiva,* which also covers the inner surface of the *eyelids.* The eyeball is moved by six *extrinsic* (outside) muscles: *superior rectus, inferior rectus, lateral rectus, medial rectus, superior oblique,* and *inferior oblique.* The front surface of the eyeball is constantly washed by a small stream of tears produced by a *lacrimal gland* situated above the eye near the

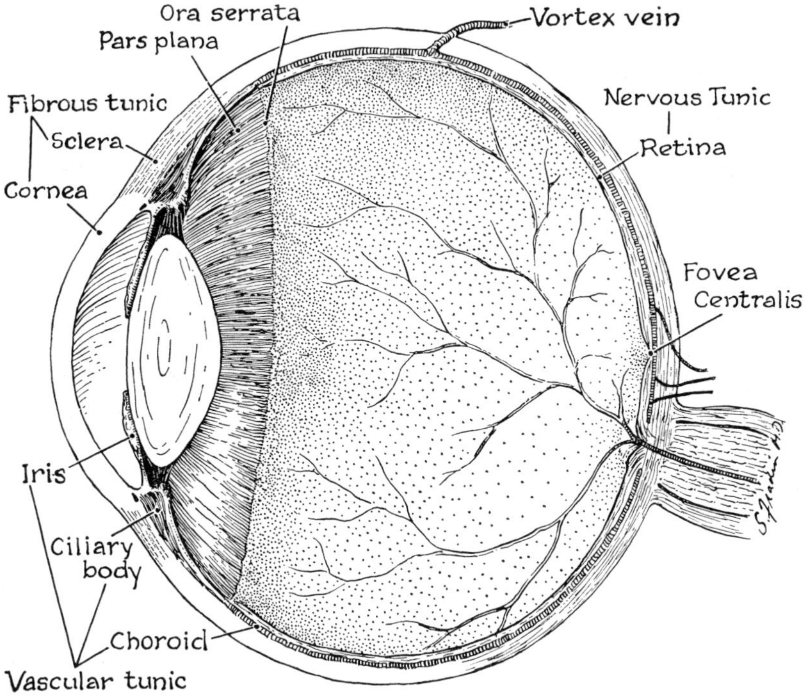

Figure 142. Diagrammatic section of the eyeball showing the delicate structures. Note the ciliary body, which controls the thickness of the lens and hence its optical power.

outer side. The excess fluid is drained from the eye by the *nasolacrimal duct* into the nose. (The conjunctiva covers only the front part of the eyeball.)

Accommodation: To obtain clear vision, the image of an object must be focused sharply on the retina. This is accomplished by the crystalline lens which must constantly change its thickness (depending on the distance of the object from the eye). The adjustment of the lens with regard to its thickness is called *accommodation*. In spite of such adjustments (controlled by the ciliary muscles), the image may not fall on the retina in good focus. This may happen when the lens is defective or the eyeball is too short or too long. If the eyeball is too short and

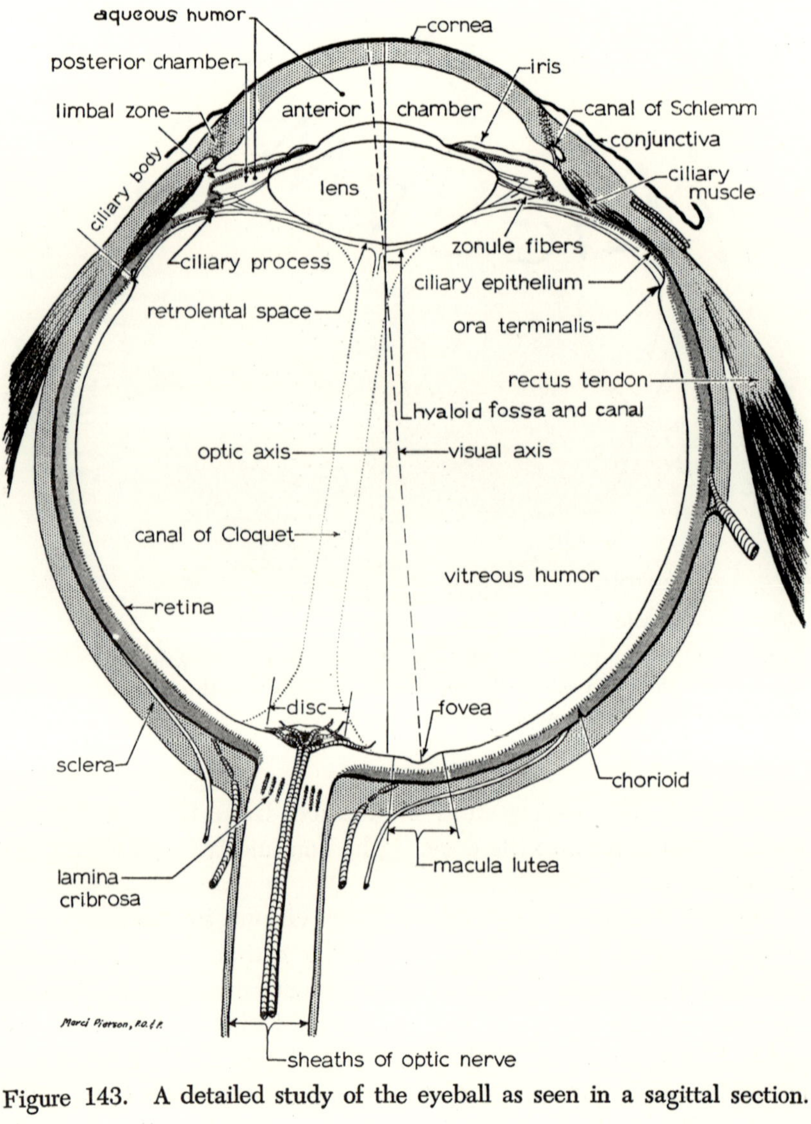

Figure 143. A detailed study of the eyeball as seen in a sagittal section.

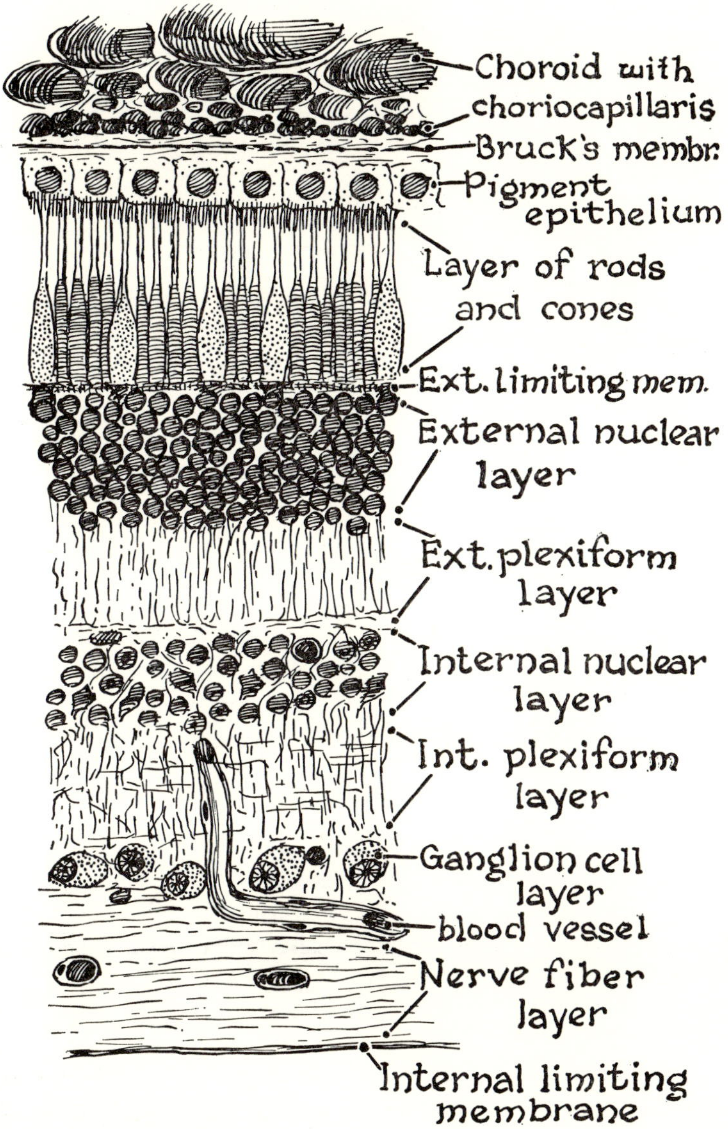

Figure 144. Microscopic study of a cross-section of the retina, showing the complexity of its structure.

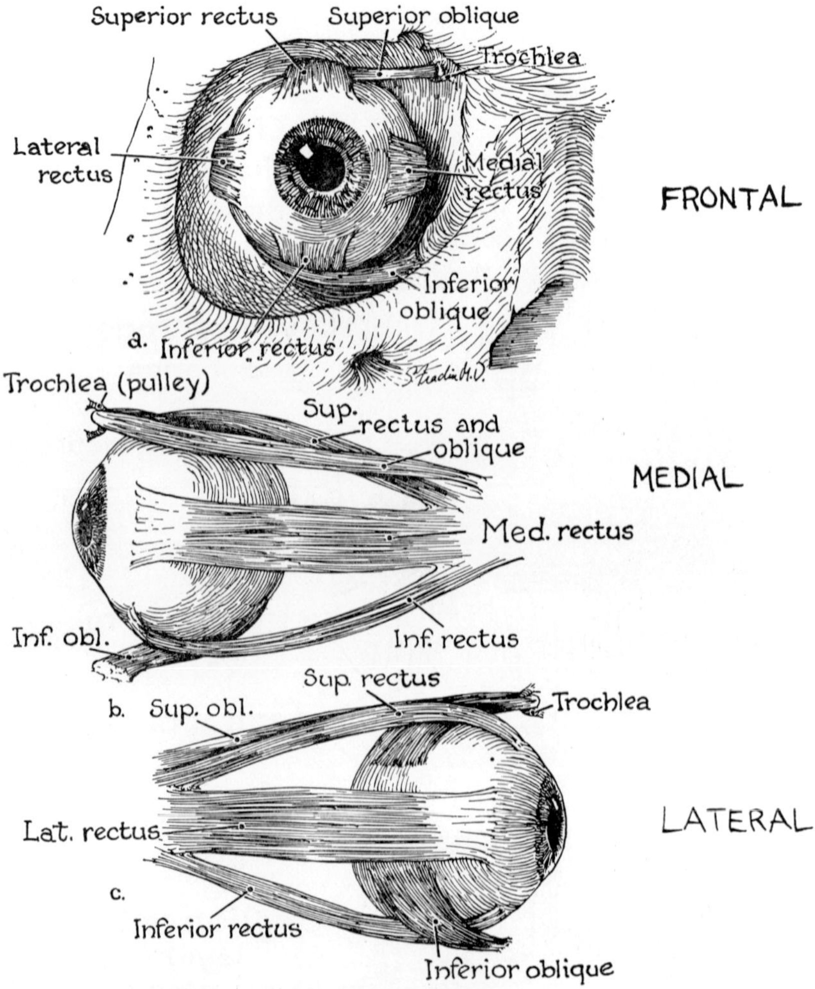

Figure 145. Three aspects of the eyeball (frontal, medial, and lateral), showing the muscles which move it in the orbit.

the rays of light are focused behind the retina, blurred vision results and the condition is known as *hyperopia* or *farsightedness*. *Convex* lenses are used to correct the situation. If the eyeball is too long or the lens is too thick in the center, the rays of light will focus in front of the retina. This is known as *myopia* or *nearsightedness*. *Concave* lenses correct myopia.

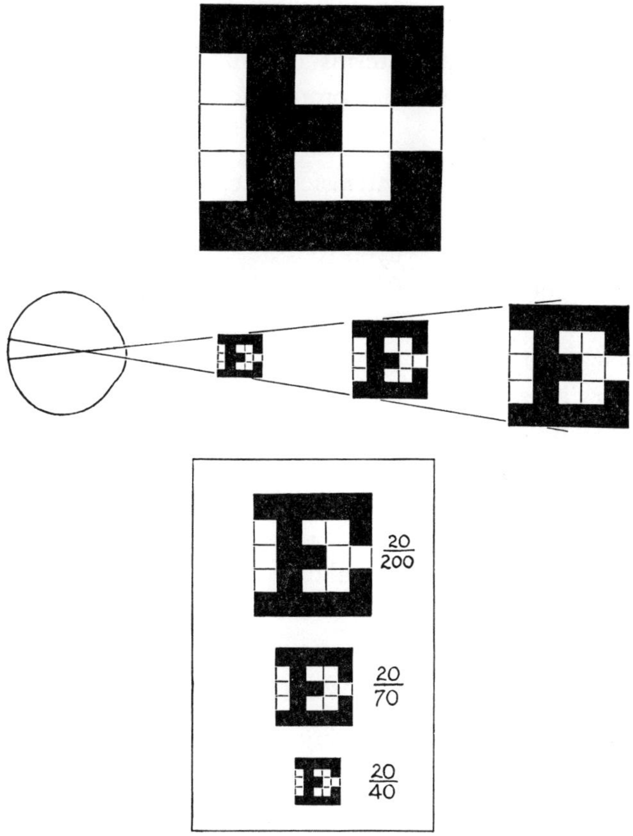

Figure 146. Snellen test type for measuring visual acuity.

VOCABULARY REVIEW

Define the following terms on the basis of the preceding discussion. Determine the pronunciation with the aid of a medical dictionary.

accommodation	extrinsic muscles	myopia
anterior chamber	eye socket	nasolacrimal duct
aqueous humor	eyelids	nearsightedness
blind spot	farsightedness	optic disk
choroid	fovea centralis	optic nerve
ciliary body	hyperopia	orbit
ciliary muscle	inferior oblique	posterior chamber
ciliary process	inferior rectus	pupil
concave	iris	retina
conjunctiva	lacrimal gland	sclera
convex	lateral rectus	superior oblique
cornea	macula lutea	superior rectus
crystalline lens	medial rectus	vitreous humor

REVIEW EXERCISE

1. Name the three layers forming the wall of the eyeball.
2. What part of the eye is the *cornea*?
3. What structure supports the crystalline lens of the eye?
4. What forms the optic disk?
5. What is the region of sharpest vision called?
6. Name the chambers of the eyeball.
7. Designate the locations of the *aqueous humor* and *vitreous humor*.
8. Name the six extrinsic muscles of the eye.

Chapter XV

THE ENDOCRINE SYSTEM

GENERAL CONSIDERATIONS. Glands which deliver their secretions to a nearby surface by means of a duct, such as a salivary gland, are known as *exocrine glands.* Glands that have no ducts and whose secretions are distributed by the blood are known as *endocrine glands.* The endocrine system is composed of the various endocrine glands, namely the *pituitary gland, thyroid gland, parathyroid glands, pancreas, adrenal glands, ovaries,* and *testes.*

The Pituitary Gland: The pituitary gland (also known as the *hypophysis* and *pituitary body*) is situated in a saddle-like hollow at the base or underside of the brain. It is divided into an *anterior lobe* and a *posterior lobe.* The anterior lobe secretes a variety of hormones: an *adrenotropic* hormone that affects the adrenal glands; a *thyrotropic* hormone affecting the thyroid gland; a *gonadotropic* hormone having an influence on the *gonads,* the testes or the ovaries; and a *growth hormone* or *somatotropic hormone* which affects body growth. Excessive growth hormone in childhood results in *gigantism* or *acromegaly.* A diminished amount of the hormone results in *dwarfism.* The posterior lobe of the pituitary gland produces *oxytocin* (which acts on the smooth muscle of the uterus), *vasopressin* (which acts on the walls of blood vessels), and an *antidiuretic* hormone (which affects the water balance of the body).

The Thyroid Gland: This gland is located in the front part of the neck. The hormone produced is called *thyroxin.* It stimulates metabolism. Excessive activity of the thyroid results in a condition called *hyperthyroidism;* insufficiency results in *hypothyroidism.*

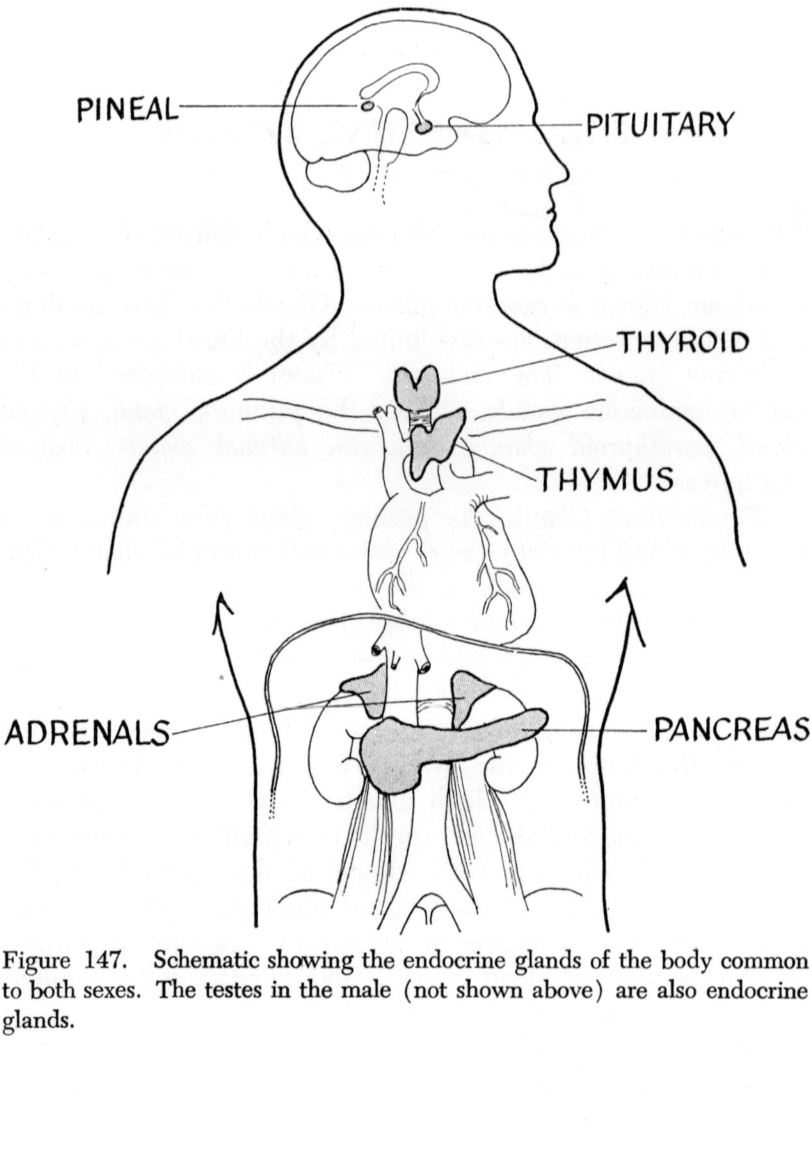

Figure 147. Schematic showing the endocrine glands of the body common to both sexes. The testes in the male (not shown above) are also endocrine glands.

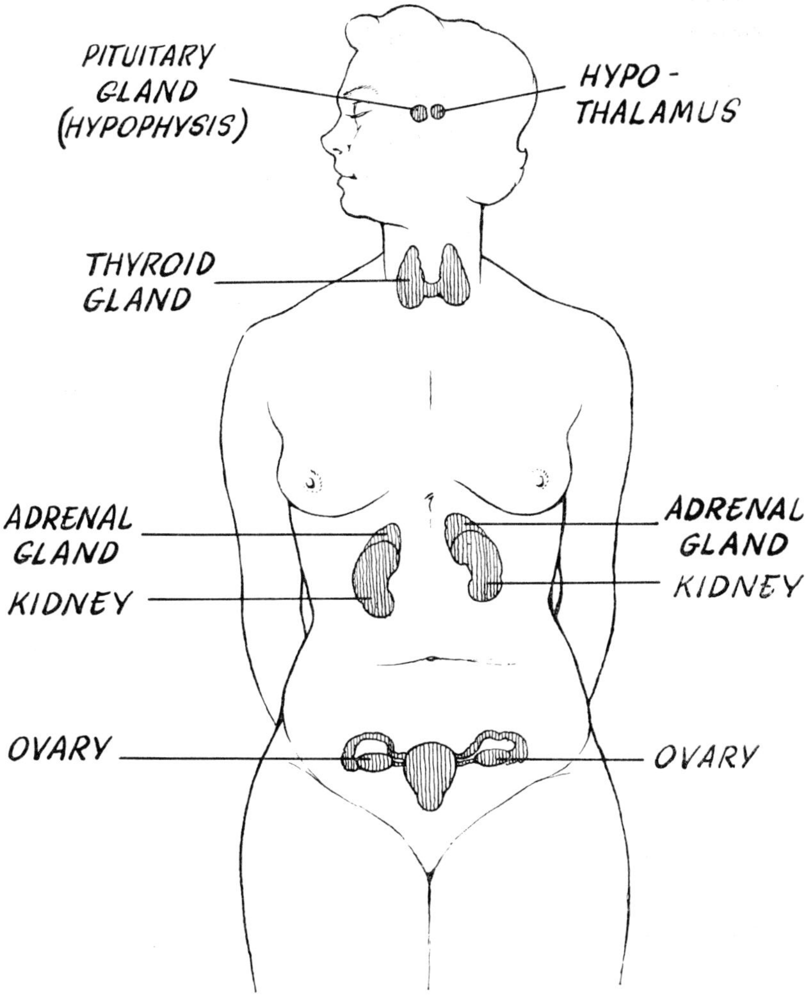

Figure 148. Schematic drawing of the endocrine glands of the female.

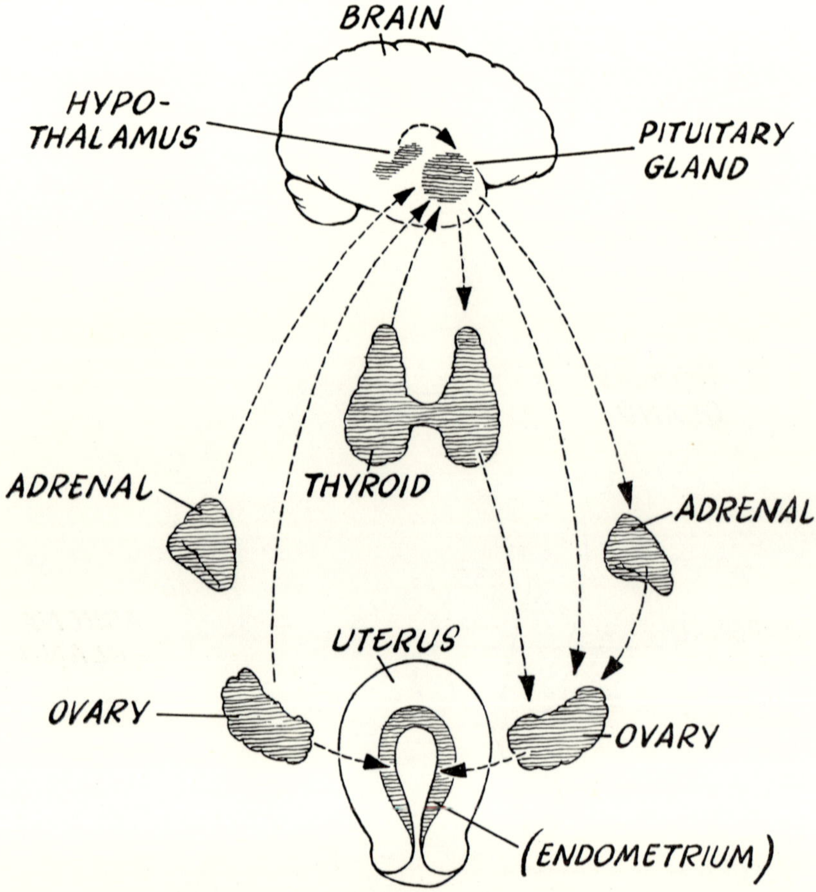

Figure 149. Diagrammatic sketch showing the functional interrelationship of the endocrine glands involved in a menstrual cycle.

Parathyroid Glands: These small glands, four to eight in number, lie on the posterior surface of the thyroid. They produce *parathormone,* which affects the metabolism of calcium and phosphorus. A deficiency in parathormone lowers the amount of calcium and phosphorus in the blood and may result in *tetany,* a spasm of muscles. Too much parathormone may lead to improper development or fragility of the bones.

The Pancreas: The pancreas lies in the abdomen, behind the

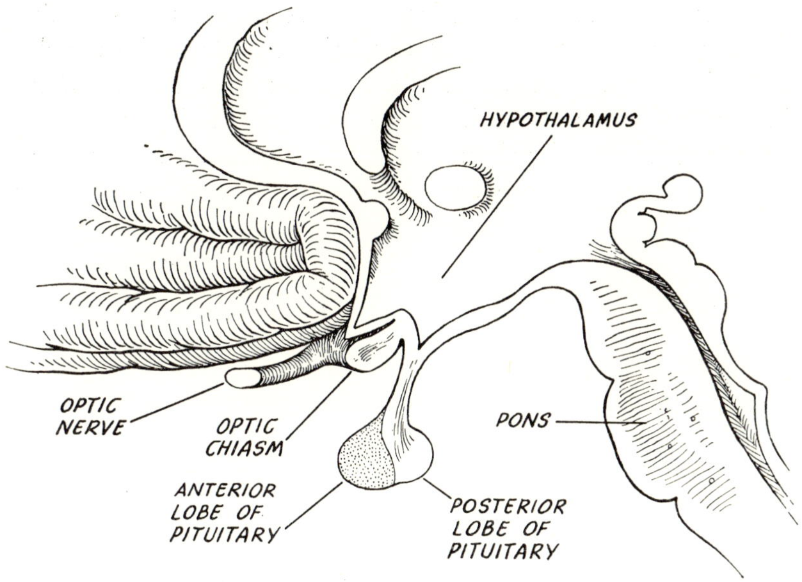

Figure 150. Diagram showing the pituitary gland in relation to the surrounding structures.

stomach. Its hormone, *insulin,* affects metabolism, especially of carbohydrates. An insufficiency of insulin may result in *diabetes mellitus,* a condition marked by *hyperglycemia* (excessive sugar in the blood) and *glycosuria* (presence of sugar in the urine). Excessive production of insulin results in *hyperinsulinism,* a condition marked by *hypoglycemia* (an abnormal decrease in the amount of sugar in the blood).

Adrenal Glands: These glands are also called *suprarenal glands.* There is one gland on the top of each kidney. Each gland is composed of a central portion, the *medulla,* and an outer part, the *cortex.* The medulla produces the hormone *epinephrine,* which has many important functions. The cortex produces a number of *corticoids,* which are chemically *steroids.* The hormones of the adrenal cortex are essential to life. They regulate the behavior of the salts and water of the body, they control metabolism, and they affect sexual development.

Ovaries and Testes: These glands of reproduction are also

known as the *gonads.* Aside from the sperm, the testes produce the male sex hormone *testosterone,* which controls the development of the sex organs and the secondary sex characteristics. The ovaries produce the hormones *estrogen* and *progesterone,* which control the development of the female sex organs, the secondary sex characteristics, and the function of menstruation.

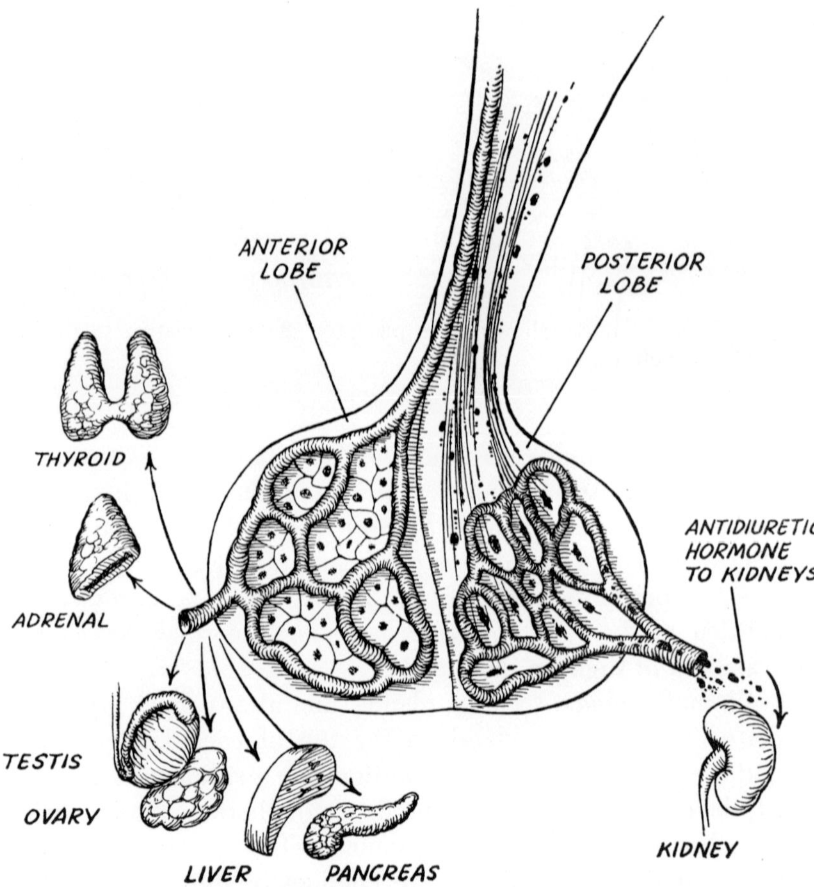

Figure 151. Diagram showing the distribution of the hormones from the anterior lobe of the pituitary gland to other glands and structures, and the effect of the posterior lobe on the function of the kidneys.

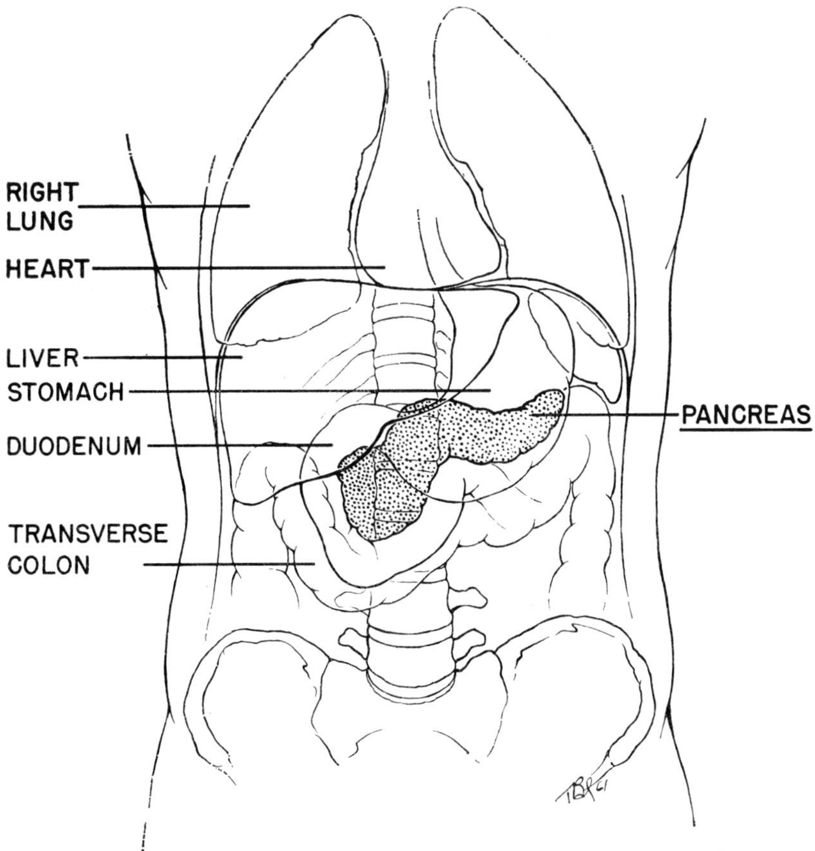

Figure 152. Diagram showing the pancreas in relation to other abdominal structures.

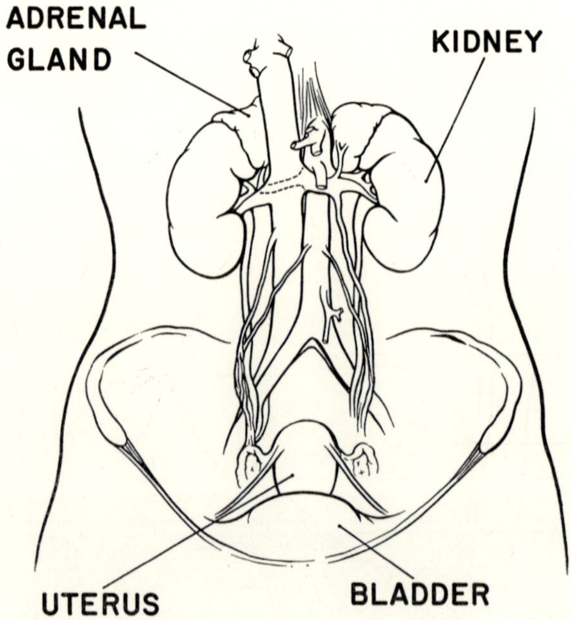

Figure 153. Drawing showing the adrenal glands in relation to the kidneys and other nearby structures.

VOCABULARY REVIEW

Define the following terms on the basis of the preceding discussion. Determine the pronunciation with the aid of a medical dictionary.

acromegaly	exocrine glands	hypothyroidism
adrenal glands	gigantism	insulin
adrenotropic	glycosuria	medulla
anterior lobe	gonadotropic	ovaries
cortex	gonads	oxytocin
corticoids	growth hormone	pancreas
diabetes mellitus	hyperglycemia	parathormone
dwarfism	hyperinsulinism	parathyroid glands
endocrine glands	hyperthyroidism	pituitary body
epinephrine	hypoglycemia	pituitary gland
estrogen	hypophysis	posterior lobe

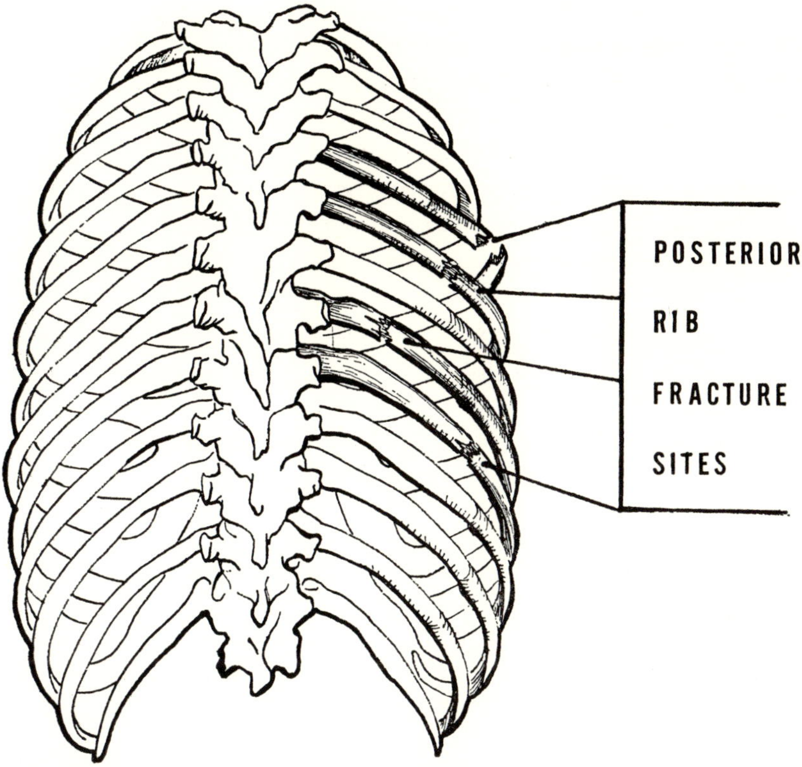

Figure 154. Diagram shows posterior view of the chest or rib cage and the sites of common rib fractures. The most commonly involved ribs are the sixth, seventh, eighth, and ninth.

progesterone	testes	thyrotropic
somatotropic	testosterone	thyroxin
steroids	tetany	vasopressin
suprarenal glands	thyroid gland	

REVIEW QUESTIONS

1. What is *acromegaly* and what causes it?
2. What are the structural components of *adrenotropic*?
3. What is the name of the tissue lying under a *cortex*?
4. Differentiate between *endocrine* and *exocrine* glands.

5. Give the meaning of *-tropic* in *gonadotropic.*
6. Give the function and location of the adrenal glands.
7. What are the components of the word *epinephrine*?
8. Give the structural units of *glycosuria.*
9. What tissue covers the *medulla* of an organ?
10. What gland or glands produce *parathormone*?
11. Locate the *pituitary gland* and name its parts.
12. What is *somatotropic* composed of?
13. Where is the *thyroid gland* located and what does it secrete?
14. Give two other names for the *hypophysis.*
15. What is the male counterpart of the female *ovaries*?
16. Name the exocrine and endocrine secretions of the *pancreas.*
17. How many *parathyroid glands* are there?
18. Give function of the *adrenal cortex hormones.*
19. What is the general term for both ovaries and testes?

Chapter XVI

ILLUSTRATIONS OF COMMON FRACTURES

THE FOLLOWING ILLUSTRATIONS show some common fractures and the methods used in their treatment: 154, 155, 156, 157, 158, 159, 160, 161, 162, 163, 164, 165.

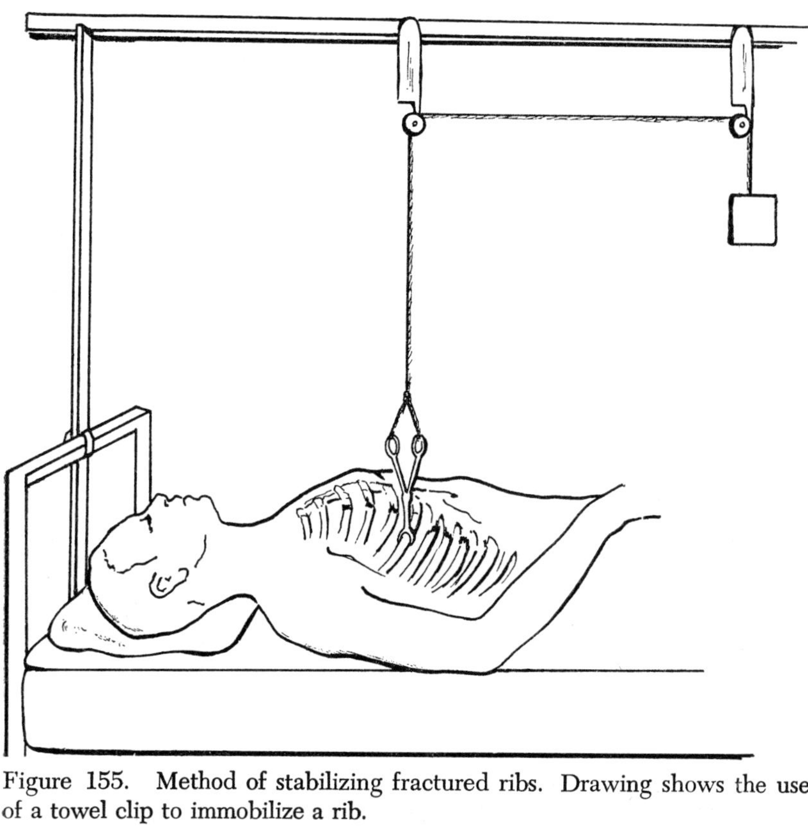

Figure 155. Method of stabilizing fractured ribs. Drawing shows the use of a towel clip to immobilize a rib.

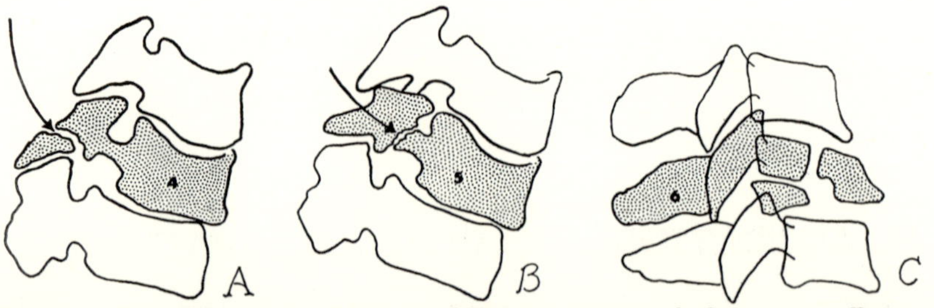

Figure 156. Schematic showing different types of fractures affecting vertebrae. *A* shows a fracture of an inferior facet. *B* shows a fracture of a vertebral arch. *C* represents a fracture of the body of the vertebra.

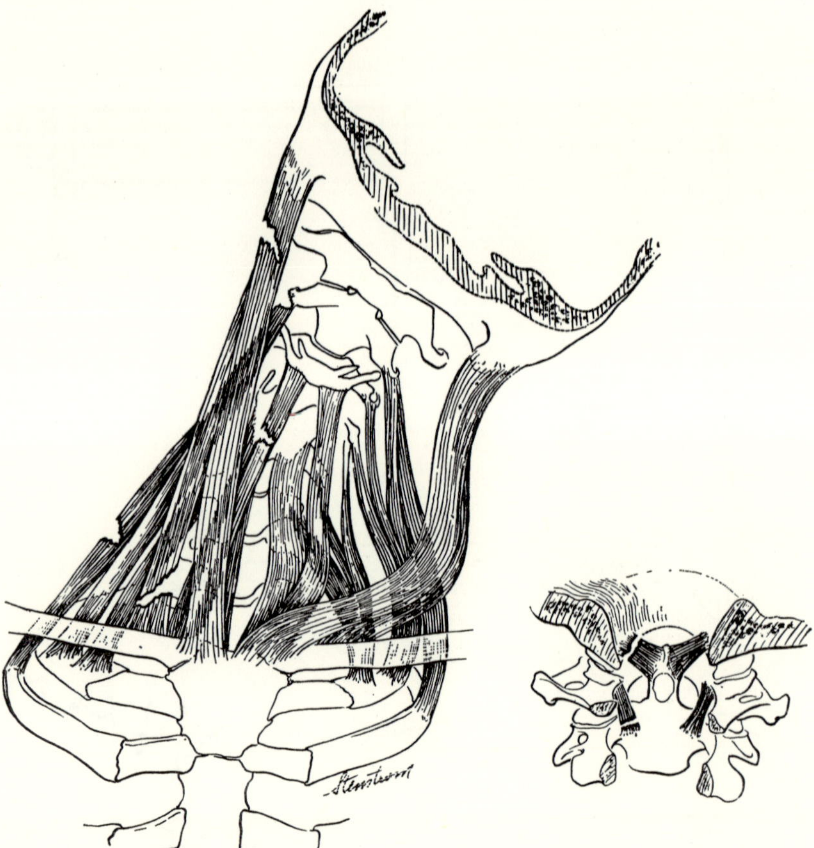

Figure 157. Drawing shows torn muscles and ligaments resulting from a violent lateral flexion and rotation of the head.

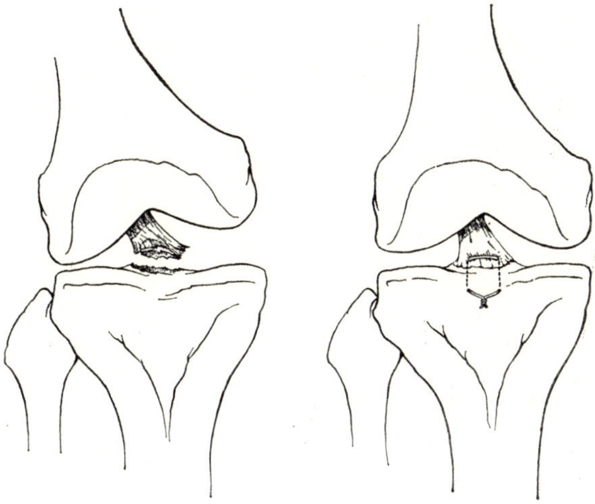

Figure 158. Drawing at left shows a rupture of the anterior cruciate ligament of the knee joint. A piece of the bone may be pulled off. Drawing at right shows the result of an arthrotomy (a cutting into the joint) in which the displaced fragment of bone is secured by a suture.

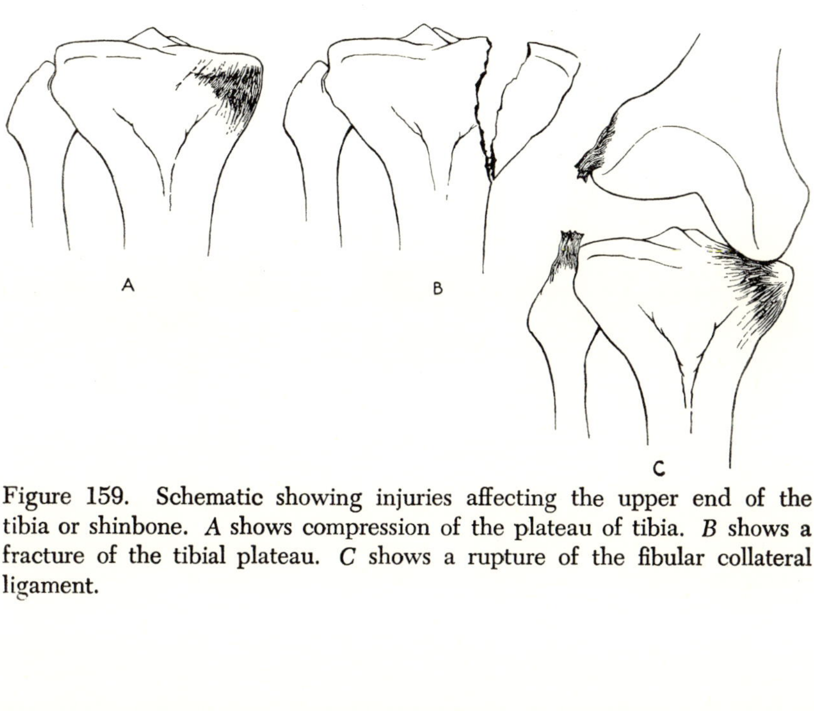

Figure 159. Schematic showing injuries affecting the upper end of the tibia or shinbone. *A* shows compression of the plateau of tibia. *B* shows a fracture of the tibial plateau. *C* shows a rupture of the fibular collateral ligament.

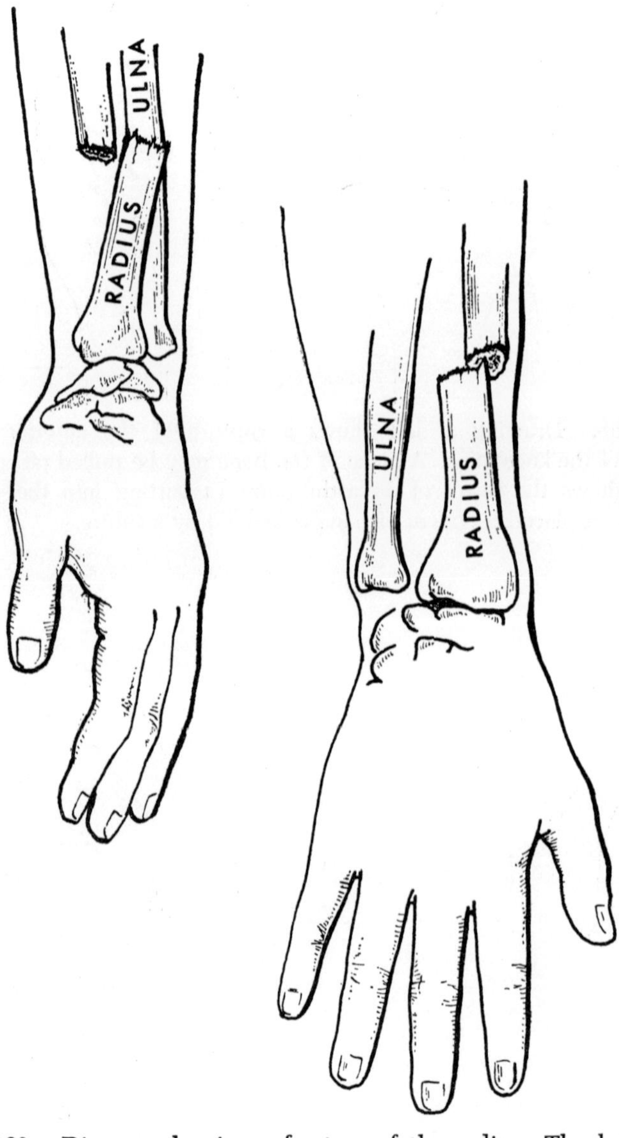

Figure 160. Diagram showing a fracture of the radius. The lower fragment is displaced toward the ulna.

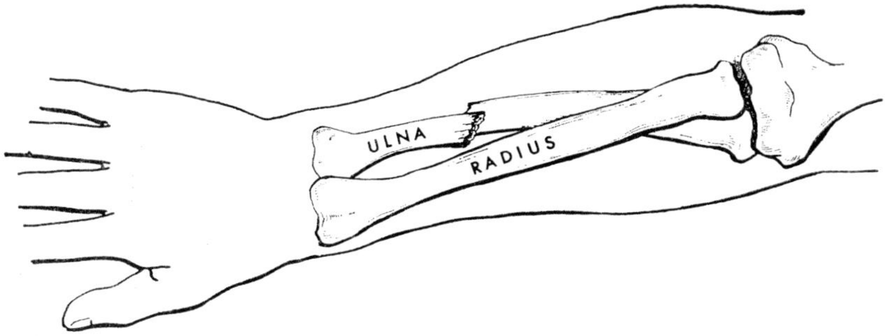

Figure 161. Diagrammatic sketch showing a fracture of the ulna.

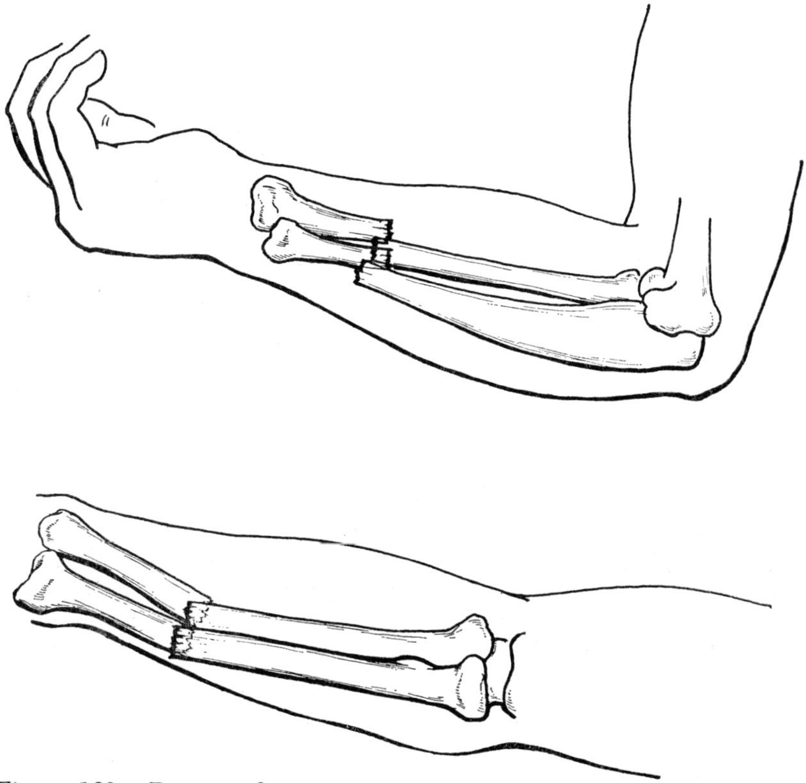

Figure 162. Diagram showing fractures of both the radius and ulna, the bones of the forearm. The upper drawing shows the position of the bone fragments while the arm is in flexion. The lower sketch shows the position while the arm is extended.

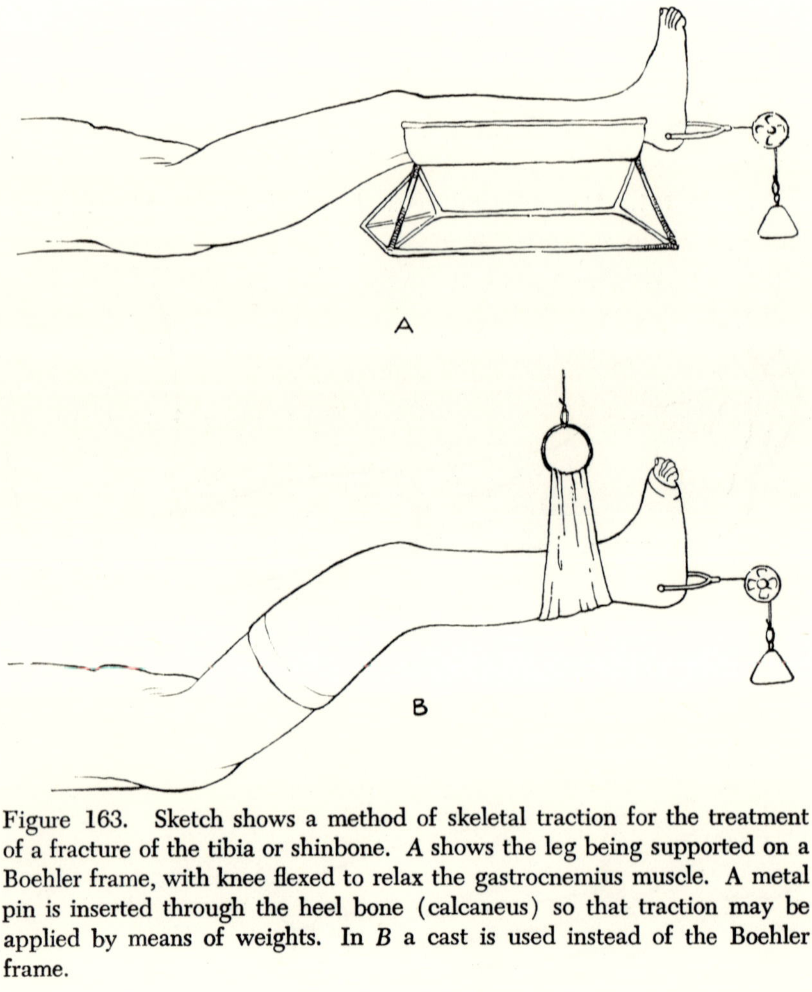

Figure 163. Sketch shows a method of skeletal traction for the treatment of a fracture of the tibia or shinbone. *A* shows the leg being supported on a Boehler frame, with knee flexed to relax the gastrocnemius muscle. A metal pin is inserted through the heel bone (calcaneus) so that traction may be applied by means of weights. In *B* a cast is used instead of the Boehler frame.

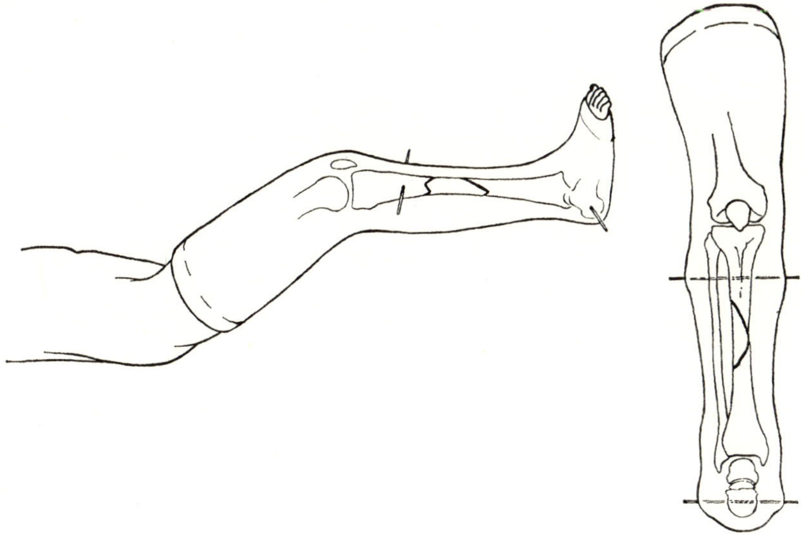

Figure 164. Two views of a technique of pins and plaster. A metal pin is inserted into the heel bone and another pin is inserted in the bone above the fracture. While traction is applied, the leg is covered by a long cast incorporating the pins. When the traction is released by removing the weight, it is still maintained by the pins in the plaster.

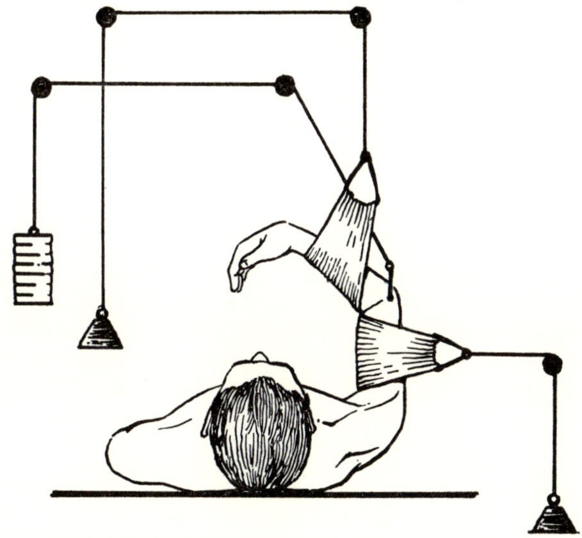

Figure 165. Diagram shows treatment of a comminuted fracture of the elbow. A pin is inserted through the olecranon of the ulna and traction is applied.